MW01382806

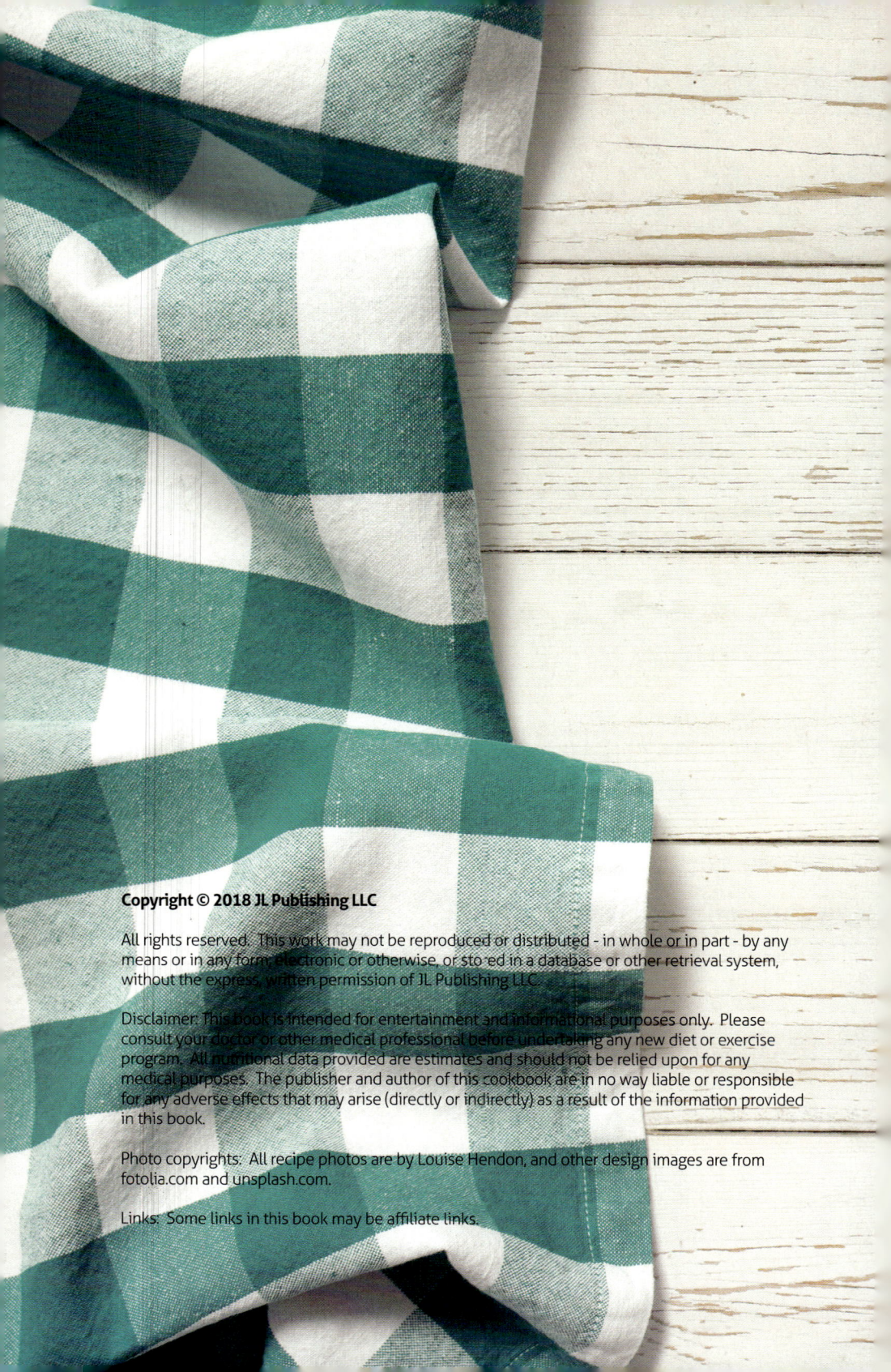

TABLE OF CONTENTS

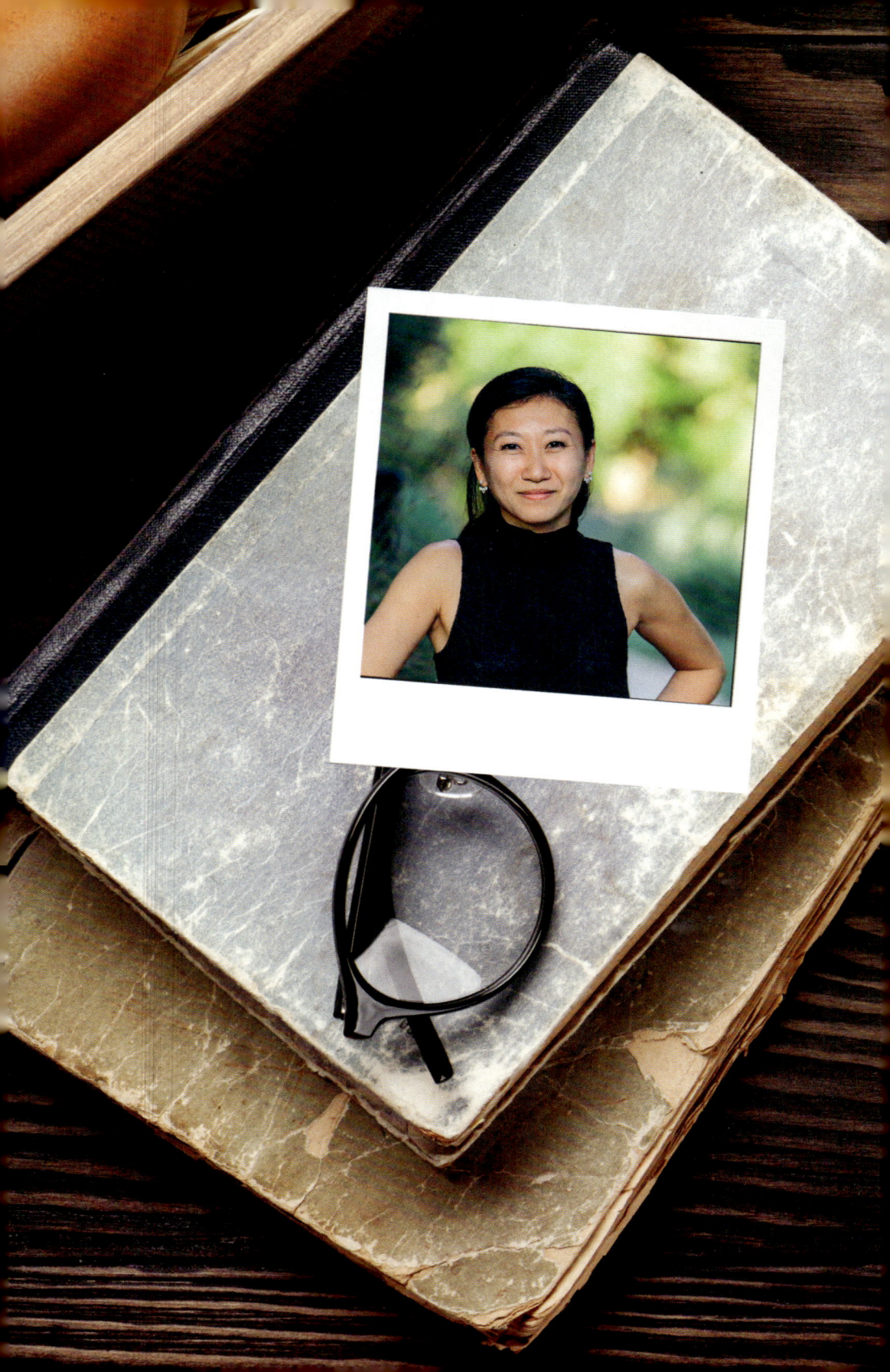

Hi! I'm Louise, the co-founder of the Keto Summit.

And I created this cookbook to help you enjoy delicious snacks without falling off the wagon.

Because I know what a struggle it can be to stay on Keto when you're traveling, working long hours, or faced with cravings at night.

Even though you love the feeling of being in ketosis - the energy, the better-fitting clothes, the positive moods, the clarity of mind, the weight-loss...

It can still be so tempting at times to fall back on old habits and grab a chocolate bar or brownie or potato chips.

Because supermarkets and restaurants simply aren't designed with your health in mind. They place the pastries where you can smell them as soon as you walk in and the candies to catch you when you're checking out.

That's why you have to plan ahead to prevent yourself from falling off the Keto wagon.

And one of the best ways to avoid cheating on your Keto diet is to arm yourself with delicious and filling Keto snacks so that you won't be tempted to grab that tub of ice-cream or pull open that packet of cookies.

All the snack recipes in this cookbook are designed to fit a low-inflammatory, low-carb, dairy-free, Paleo, and Keto lifestyle. So you can enjoy these delicious snacks without feeling bloated, guilty, and berating yourself for your lack of persistence the next day.

The journey to long-lasting health and staying slim and fit isn't always easy. But you can make it easier for yourself by planning ahead and knowing where your weaknesses lie.

For example, if you turn to potato chips when you're stressed or popcorn when you watch movies or ice-cream when you're sad, then pick out Keto versions of these foods from this cookbook.

Print out your favorite go-to emergency snack recipes and stick them on your fridge door for when temptation comes.

Or make a large batch of the peppermint patties and store them in your freezer.

Be prepared so that you can Keto on to long-lasting

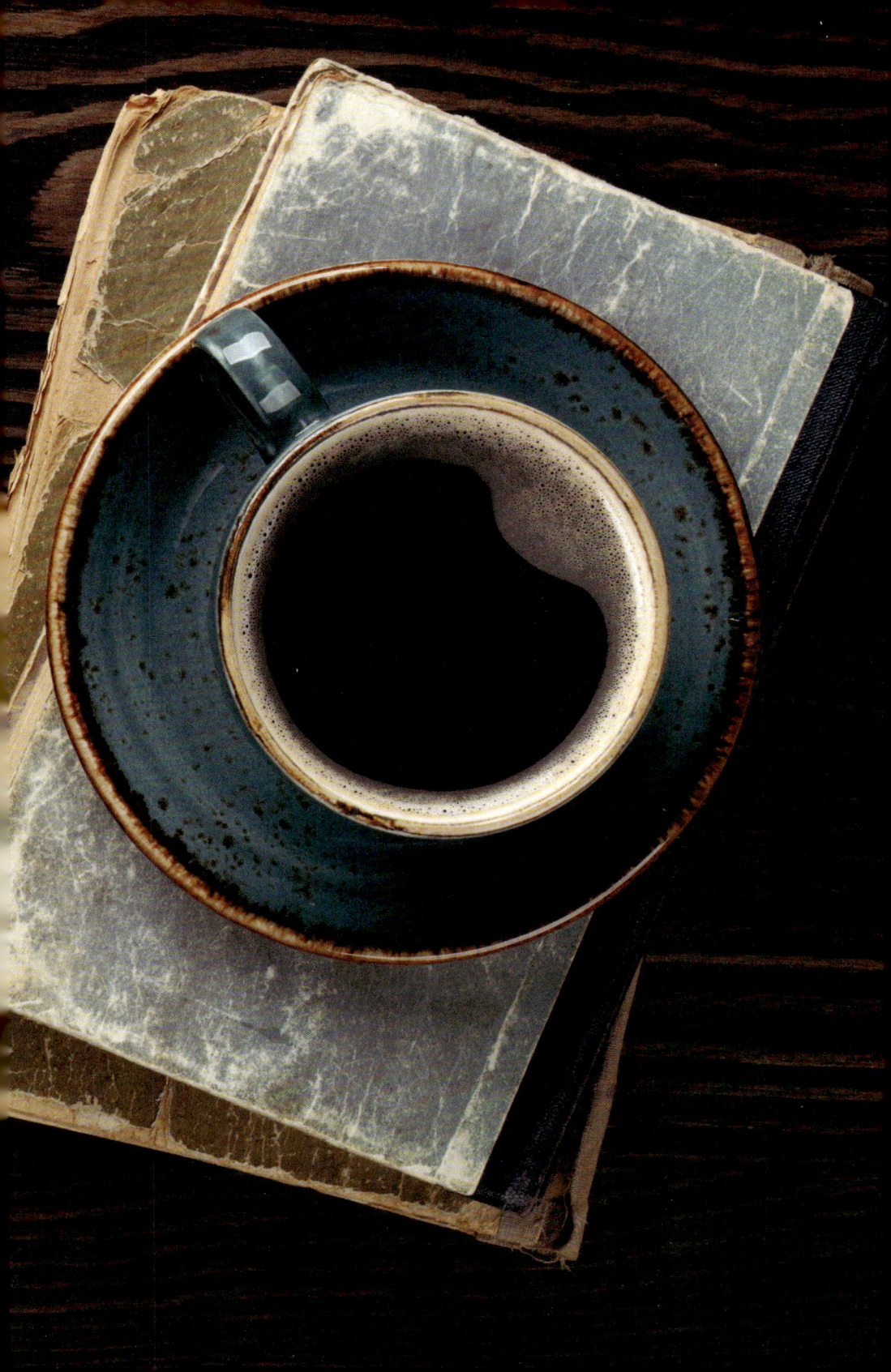

How To Use

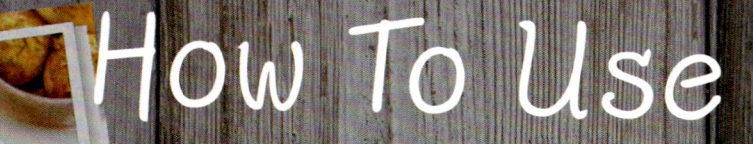

1

All recipes have yields so please check the number of servings carefully so you don't overeat these snacks.

2

This book is interactive, so you can click on links to jump between sections easily. Some blue links go to websites like amazon.com or to additional recipes.

3

There are 59 recipes in this book, and you can pick and choose whichever snacks fit your mood and lifestyle.

4

Nutritional information (calories, total fat, net carbohydrates, and protein) has been provided for each recipe. Please note that these are just estimates. (Net Carbohydrates = Total Carbohydrates minus Fiber)

This Book

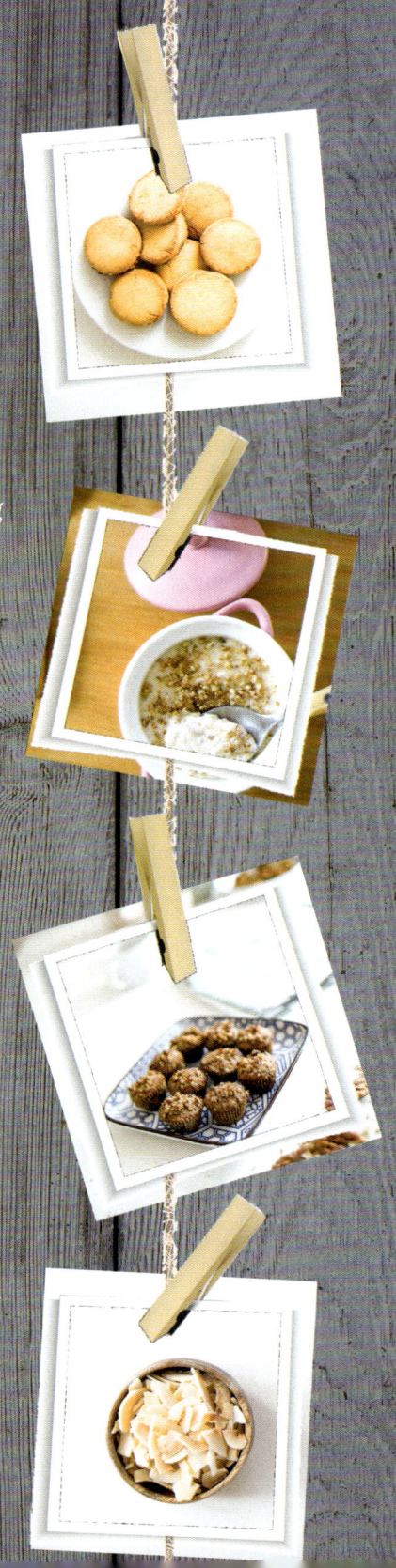

5

These snacks should not form the basis of your Keto diet! Just remember that these are for when you're traveling, craving something sweet, or have a party.

6

I'm a big fan of batch cooking and cooking in advance. And many of the snacks are great for this...like the Peppermint Patties, Pecan Crisps, and Cajun Roasted Almonds.

7

If you have any questions about the recipes in this cookbook, then please email me at louise@ketosummit.com and I'll try to reply as quickly as possible.

8

Cooking and learning how to heal and nourish your body is all part of the Keto journey. So please enjoy!

easy, no~cook

Idea #1 - Cucumber Slices/Celery Sticks

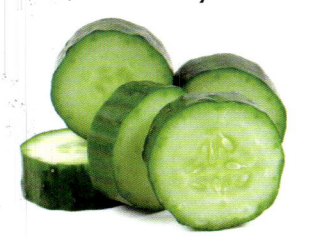

Idea #2 - Canned Tuna

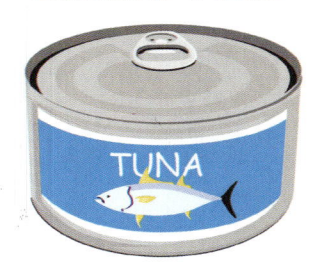

Idea #3 - Canned Sardines

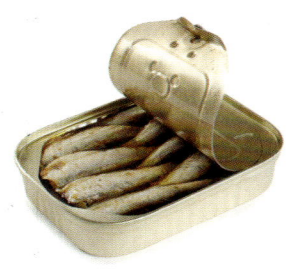

Idea #4 - Coconut Butter

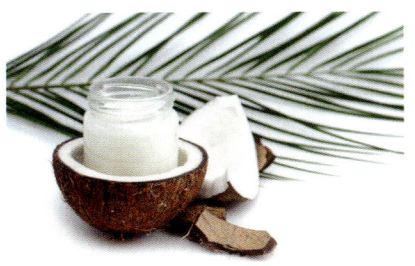

Idea #5 - 100% Chocolate

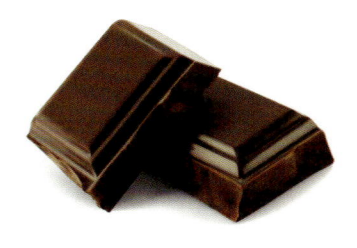

Idea #6 - Nuts & Seeds

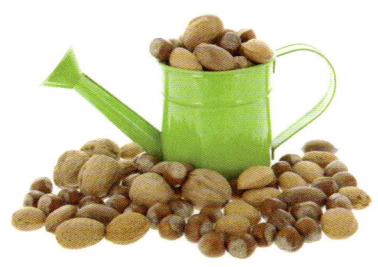

Keto snacks

Idea #7 - Avocado

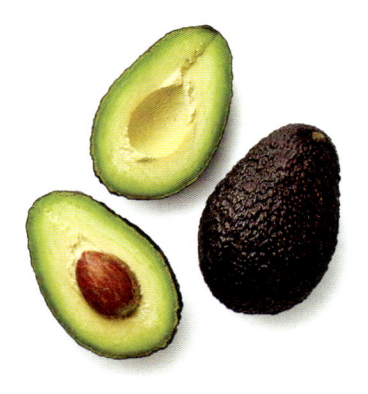

Idea #10 - Beef sticks/ Jerky

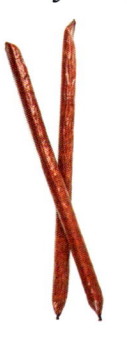

Idea #8 - Olives

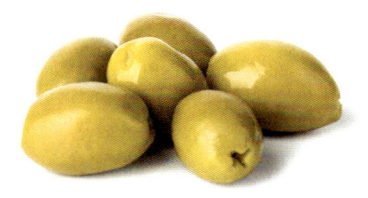

Idea #11 - Cacao Nibs

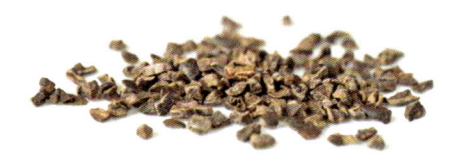

Idea #9 - Almond Butter

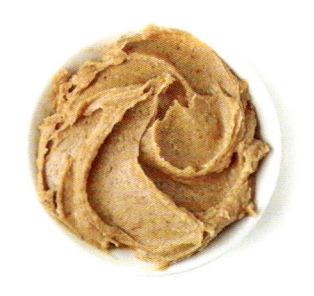

Idea #12 - Smoked Salmon/Deli Meats

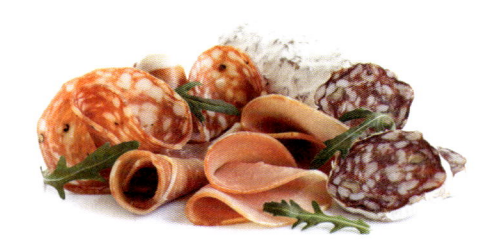

Ingredients

The focus of a good Keto diet is to help nourish your body while keeping your body in ketosis.

Green leafy vegetables, seafoods, fish, meats, and healthy fats should make up the bulk of your diet.

But there are some other ingredients that Keto snacks often use:

ALMOND FLOUR & ALMOND MEAL
Almond flour is very finely ground almonds. You can make your own almond flour by food processing whole almonds into a rough meal.

COCONUT BUTTER
Coconut butter (or coconut manna) is like almond butter but made from shredded coconut.

COCONUT FLOUR
This is finely ground de-fatted dried coconut.

COCONUT MILK
This usually comes in 2 forms, cartons or cans. The canned milk tends to be a lot thicker and higher in fat content. If you refrigerate the cans, the coconut cream rises to the top and can be scooped out. All recipes in this book uses the cans.

STEVIA

Stevia is a great Keto sweetener that typically doesn't cause any issues for people. The main downside is that it can leave a bitter aftertaste that some people dislike.

ERYTHRITOL

This is a sugar alcohol that typically causes fewer digestive issues for people. It's great for baking but don't use too much. Try mixing some erythritol with stevia.

FLAX/CHIA SEEDS

Grind these seeds to form a flour/meal that can help stick baked goods together (like eggs do). Best to use a coffee grinder and grind your own as they can go rancid quickly.

MAYO

Most mayos use canola or sunflower or other seed oils that are often rancid and highly processed. But you can make your own by using coconut oil, avocado oil, or olive oil. You can also purchase Paleo mayo in the US.

GHEE

Ghee can be made from butter. It's clarified butter. While we suggest you omit dairy on Keto to maximize your weight loss and health, ghee is typically fine as the milk proteins have been removed. You can make your own by heating butter gently until the milk solids brown and sink.

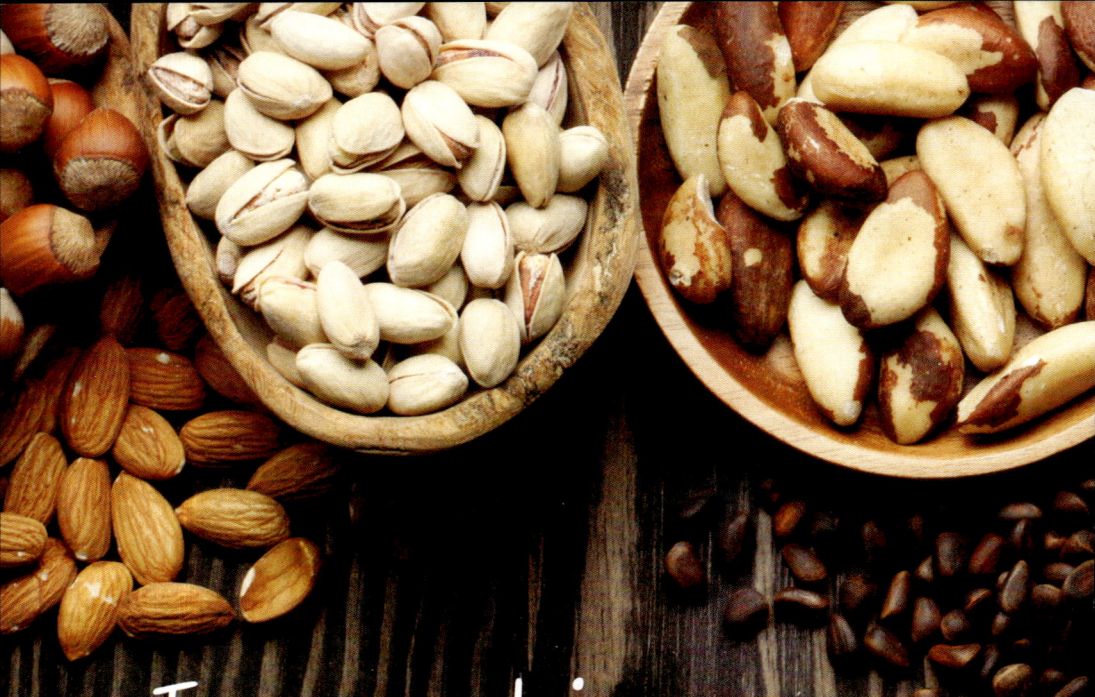

Is snacking even good on Keto?

As you are probably already aware, snacking can be a bad habit that causes overeating and relies too much on Keto sugars and nuts rather than highly nutritious foods like vegetables, meats, and seafood.

But there are several circumstances when Keto snacks can really help...

1. WHEN YOU'RE HAVING CRAVINGS

Cravings can often catch you unawares. So make sure you have healthy Keto snacks available so that you don't end up eating chocolate bars, cookies, potato chips, and whatever other junk food you might see or have handy.

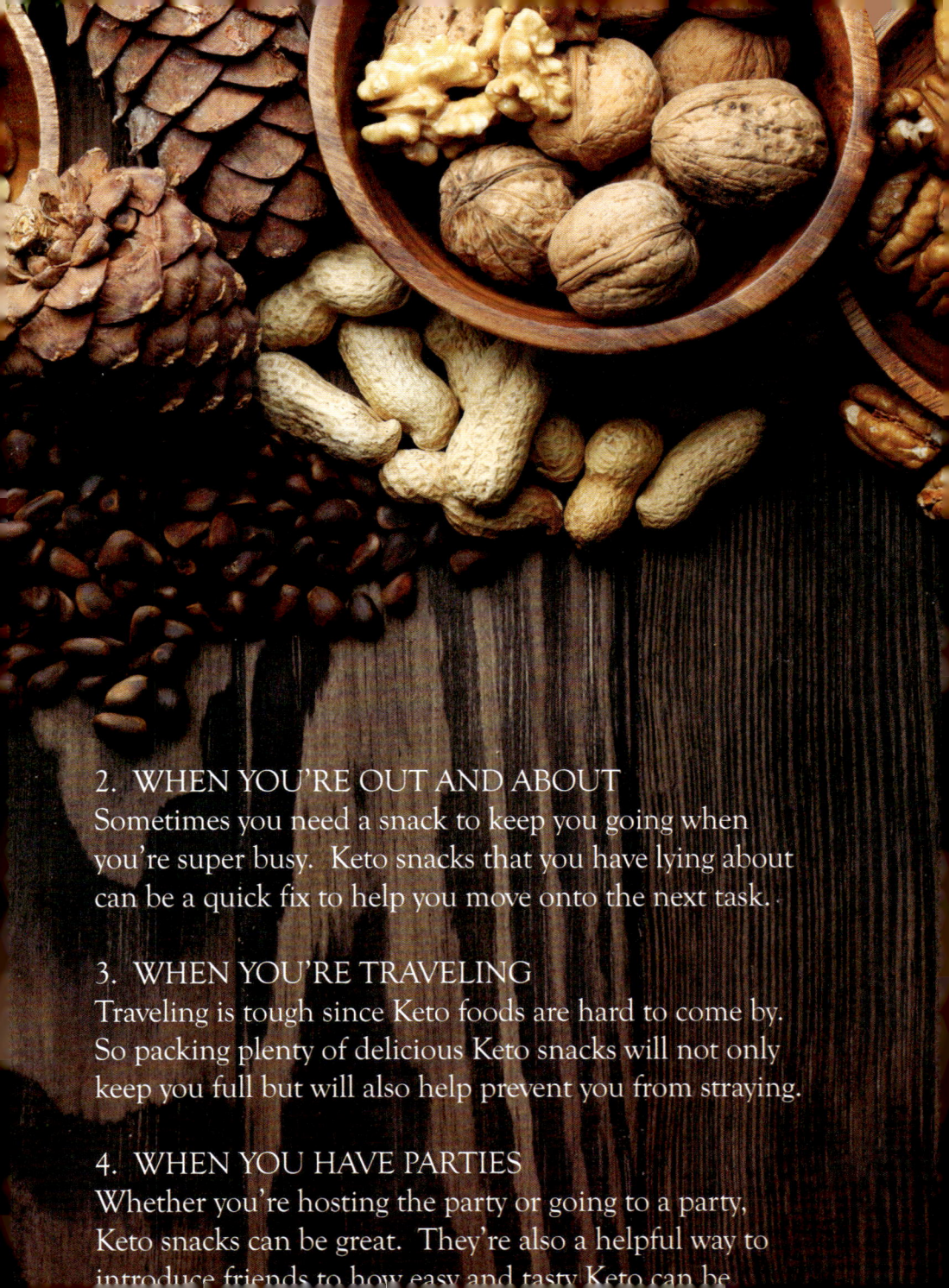

2. WHEN YOU'RE OUT AND ABOUT

Sometimes you need a snack to keep you going when you're super busy. Keto snacks that you have lying about can be a quick fix to help you move onto the next task.

3. WHEN YOU'RE TRAVELING

Traveling is tough since Keto foods are hard to come by. So packing plenty of delicious Keto snacks will not only keep you full but will also help prevent you from straying.

4. WHEN YOU HAVE PARTIES

Whether you're hosting the party or going to a party, Keto snacks can be great. They're also a helpful way to introduce friends to how easy and tasty Keto can be.

Chapter 1:

Chips and Crackers

Tortilla Chips

Prep Time: 5 minutes
Cook Time: 10 minutes
Yield: 2 servings

INGREDIENTS

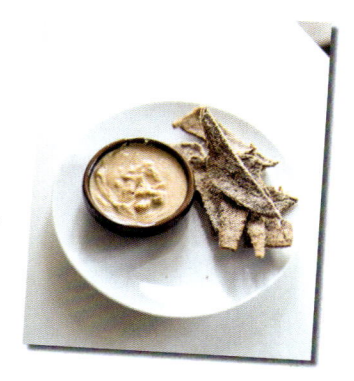

- 1/3 cup (60 g) chia or flax meal (use chia or flax seed, and use a coffee grinder or a good blender to process into a flour first)
- 1/3 cup (40 g) almond flour
- 1 Tablespoon (3 g) Italian seasoning
- 1 teaspoon (5 g) salt
- Water to combine to form a dough (approx. 2 Tablespoons or 30 ml)

INSTRUCTIONS

1. Mix all the ingredients together to form a dough.

2. Place the dough on small piece of parchment paper (so it can fit into the microwave). Place another piece of parchment paper on top and use a rolling pin to roll the dough into a thin sheet (1 mm-thick - it has to be thin so that the microwave can dry it out quickly).

3. Remove the top layer of paper and score the dough into triangles (like chips) and place the flattened dough with the parchment paper into the microwave for 2 minutes. Check on the chips to make sure they're not burning. Then cook in 1-minute segments until crispy.

4. Alternatively, you can place in a preheated oven at 300 F (150 C) for around 10 minutes (check oven to make sure the chips don't burn).

5. Or, if you have a dehydrator, then dehydrate at a low temperature for approx. 4 hours until crispy.

6. Season with salt and enjoy with one of the dips from this book.

Nutritional Data (estimates) - per serving:
Calories: 121   Fat: 9 g   Total Carbs: 8 g   Fiber: 5 g   Sugar: 0 g   Net Carbs: 3 g   Protein: 4 g

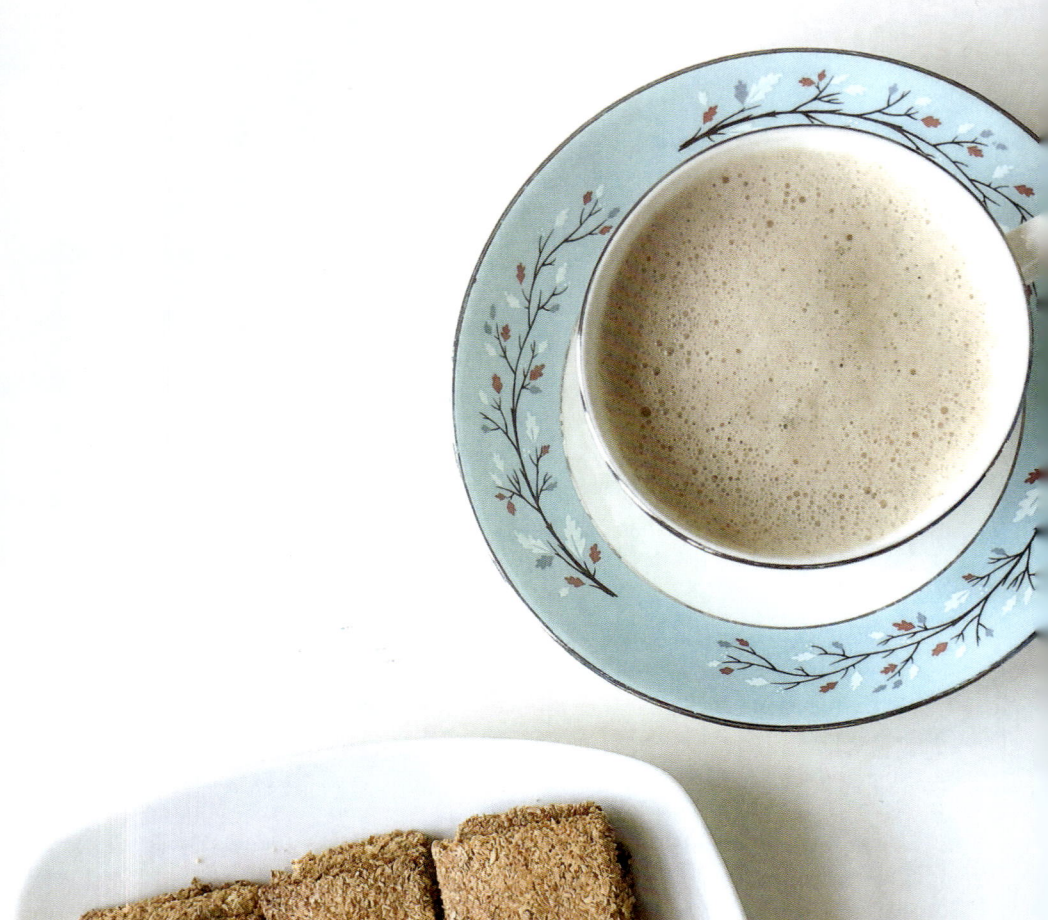
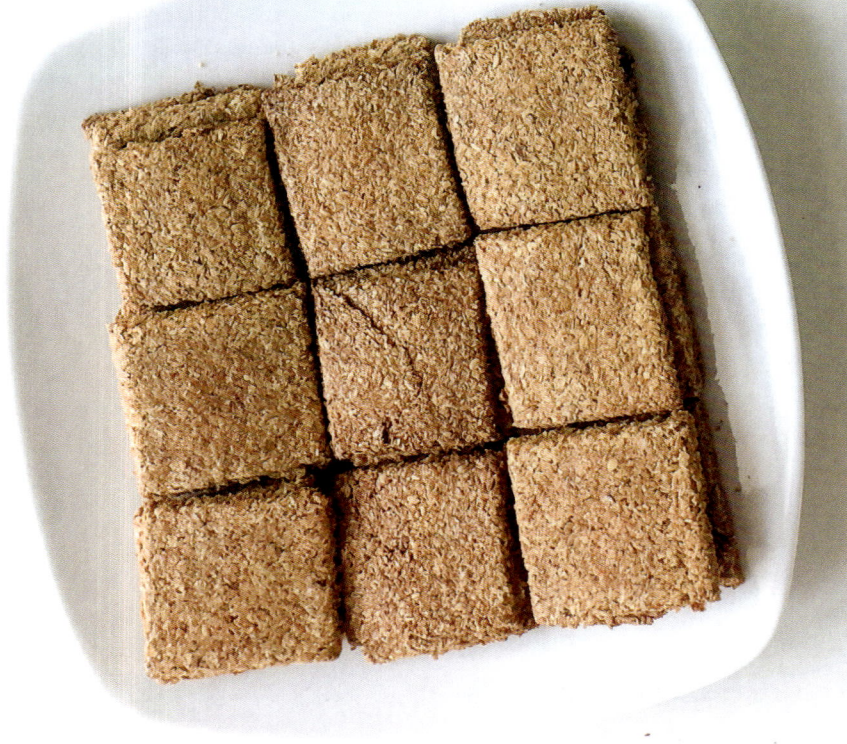

Italian Flaxseed Crackers

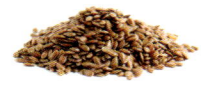

Prep Time: 15 minutes
Cook Time: 35 minutes
Yield: 4 servings

INGREDIENTS

- 1 cup (120 g) flax seeds, ground into a meal (use a food processor, blender, or coffee grinder)
- 1/2 cup (120 ml) water
- 1 Tablespoon (10 g) garlic powder
- 2 teaspoons (5 g) onion powder
- 1 Tablespoon (3 g) Italian seasoning
- 1 teaspoon (5 g) salt

INSTRUCTIONS

1. Preheat oven to 400 F (200 C).
2. In a medium mixing bowl, combine flax meal with all the other dry ingredients. Add water and stir until combined. Knead for a few minutes to form a dough.
3. Place the dough onto a large piece of parchment paper and lay on a flat surface. Place another piece of parchment paper on top of the dough.
4. Use a rolling pin to roll the dough to desired thickness (approx. 0.3 cm).
5. Gently pull the top piece of parchment paper away from the dough. Use a sharp knife or pizza cutter and score the flattened dough into square crackers.
6. Place the parchment paper with the scored dough onto a baking tray and bake for 10-15 minutes (they should be easy to lift off the parchment paper but not crunchy).
7. Carefully pull the crackers apart and flip them over.
8. Reduce oven heat to 300 F (150 C).
9. Bake for another 15-20 minutes until crispy but not burnt.
10. If you have a dehydrator, you can place the crackers in a dehydrator for 6-8 hours on low until they're not soft anymore.

Nutritional Data (estimates) - per serving:
Calories: 151 Fat: 12 g Total Carbs: 10 g Fiber: 6 g Sugar: 1 g Net Carbs: 4 g Protein: 6 g

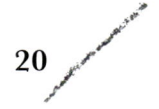

Easy Zucchini Chips

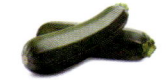

Prep Time: 2 minutes
Cook Time: 1 hour
Yield: 4 servings

INGREDIENTS

- 1 zucchini, very thinly sliced (use a mandolin if possible)
- 2 Tablespoons (30 ml) olive oil
- 1/4 teaspoon (1 g) salt

INSTRUCTIONS

1. Preheat oven to 300 F (150 C). (If your oven goes lower, then place it on a lower heat. Or use a dehydrator.)
2. Pat the zucchini slices very dry using a paper towel to soak up excess water.
3. Toss the slices with the olive oil and salt.
4. Place on a large parchment paper-lined baking tray and bake for 1 hour (it may need to be longer if you used a much lower oven temperature or a dehydrator) until the chips are crispy.

Nutritional Data (estimates) - per serving:
Calories: 64 Fat: 7 g Total Carbs: 1 g Fiber: 0 g Sugar: 1 g Net Carbs: 1 g Protein: 0 g

Toasted Coconut Flakes

Prep Time: 5 minutes
Cook Time: 7 minutes
Yield: 4 servings

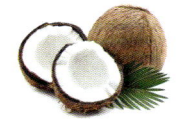

INGREDIENTS

- 2 Tablespoons (30 ml) coconut oil, slightly melted
- 1 cup (60 g) coconut flakes
- 2 Tablespoons (24 g) erythritol or stevia, to taste (optional)
- Dash of salt

INSTRUCTIONS

1. Preheat oven to 300 F (150 C).
2. Mix the coconut flakes in the coconut oil, sweetener, and salt.
3. Place on a parchment paper-lined baking tray.
4. Bake for 6-7 minutes. Remove quickly as it burns fast.
5. Let cool and enjoy.

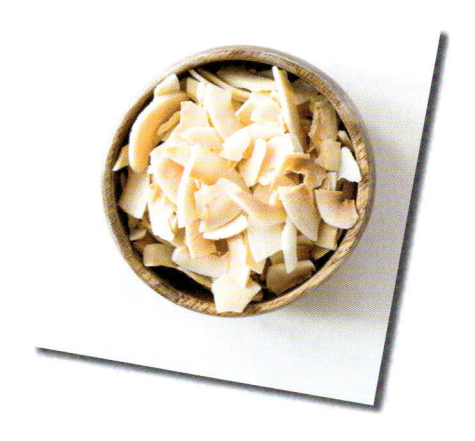

Nutritional Data (estimates) - per serving:
Calories: 172 Fat: 17 g Total Carbs: 6 g Fiber: 3 g Sugar: 1 g Net Carbs: 3 g Protein: 2 g

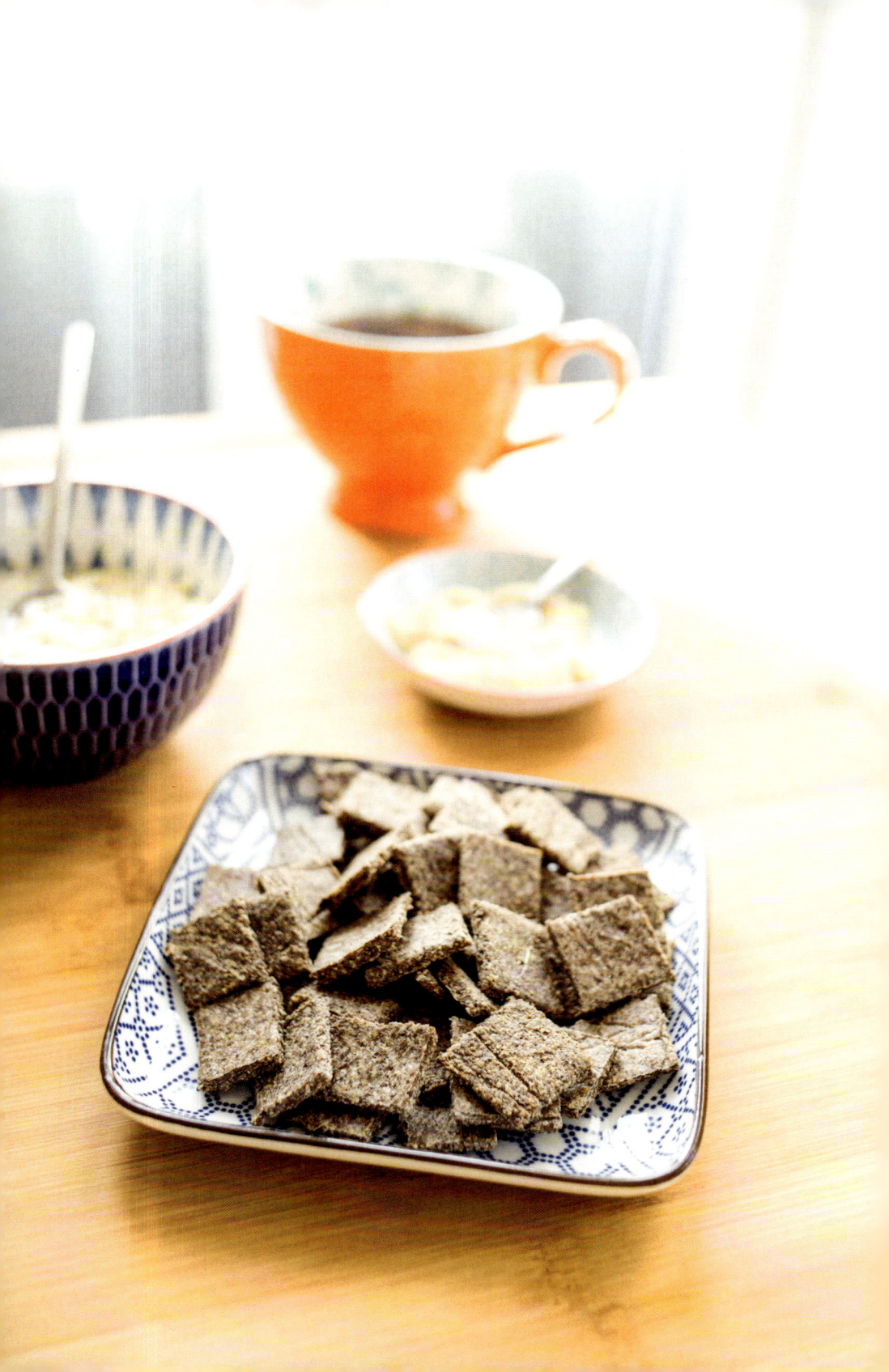

Crunchy Garlic Chia Crackers

Prep Time: 15 minutes
Cook Time: 30 minutes
Yield: 4 servings

INGREDIENTS

- 1/2 cup (60 g) chia or flax meal (use chia or flax seed, and use a coffee grinder or a good blender to process into a flour first)
- 1 egg, whisked
- 2 Tablespoons (24 g) chia seeds
- 1 Tablespoon (10 g) garlic powder
- 1 teaspoon (5 g) salt

INSTRUCTIONS

1. Preheat oven to 300 F (150 C).

2. In a mixing bowl, combine all the ingredients.

3. Place a piece of parchment paper on a flat surface. Place the dough on top of the paper and place another piece of parchment paper on top of the dough.

4. Use a rolling pin to roll the dough to desired thickness (approx. 0.1-0.2 cm thick).

5. Carefully pull the top piece of parchment paper away and use a sharp knife to score the dough into small cracker squares.

6. Place the parchment paper with the scored dough on a baking tray and bake for 15 minutes.

7. Break the crackers apart, flip the crackers over, and bake for another 15 minutes. The crackers will get harder after cooling.

8. Enjoy with the garlic dip (see recipe on page 30).

Nutritional Data (estimates) - per serving:
Calories: 123   Fat: 9 g   Total Carbs: 8 g   Fiber: 5 g   Sugar: 1 g   Net Carbs: 3 g   Protein: 6 g

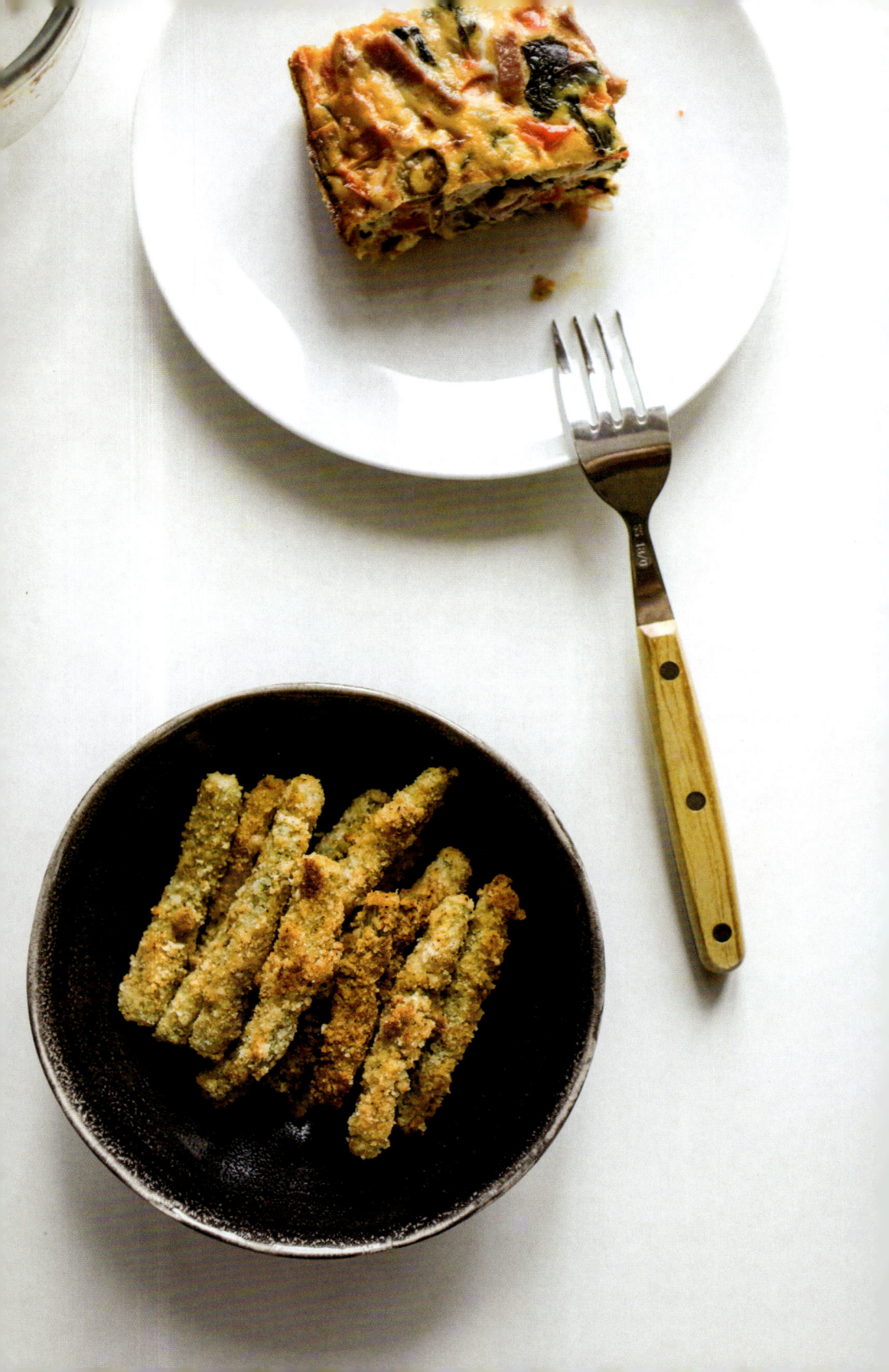

Paprika Lime Green Bean Fries

Prep Time: 10 minutes
Cook Time: 25 minutes
Yield: 4 servings

INGREDIENTS

- 1/2 lb (225 g) green beans, cut into half
- 1 egg, whisked
- 1/2 cup (60 g) almond flour or any nut flour of your choice
- 1 Tablespoon (6 g) paprika
- Zest of 1 lime
- Salt and pepper, to taste

INSTRUCTIONS

1. Preheat oven to 350 F (175 C).

2. Combine the dry ingredients (almond flour, paprika, lime zest, salt and pepper) together.

3. Dredge the green beans in the whisked egg first then generously coat with the dry mixture. It can be a bit hard to stick so press the mixture on well.

4. Place individually on a parchment paper-lined baking sheet and bake for 20-25 minutes until golden. (Note - these are not crispy fries.)

Nutritional Data (estimates) - per serving:
Calories: 107 Fat: 7 g Total Carbs: 7 g Fiber: 4 g Sugar: 1 g Net Carbs: 3 g Protein: 6 g

Cheesy Kale Chips

Prep Time: 10 minutes
Cook Time: 25 minutes
Yield: 6 servings

INGREDIENTS

- 12 oz (340 g) kale leaves (with stems on, the bag will weigh around 12 oz but with stems removed, they'll only be 7-8 oz)
- 1/2 cup (70 g) cashews
- 1/4 cup (32 g) nutritional yeast
- 4 Tablespoons (60 ml) olive oil, divided into two
- Salt and pepper, to taste

INSTRUCTIONS

1. Preheat oven to 300 F (150 C). (If your oven goes lower, then place it on a lower heat. Or use a dehydrator.)
2. Remove the stem and pat each kale leaf dry. Toss with 2 tablespoons of olive oil.
3. Place the rest of the ingredients (cashews, yeast, 2 tablespoons of olive oil, salt and pepper) into a blender and blend well.
4. Toss with the kale leaves so that the mixture sticks on them.
5. Place kale leaves on large baking trays and bake for 20-25 minutes (flip after 10 minutes). If you're baking at 300 F, then you might want to open the oven door a tiny bit to ensure the kale chips don't burn.

Nutritional Data (estimates) - per serving:
Calories: 177 Fat: 14 g Total Carbs: 9 g Fiber: 3 g Sugar: 2 g Net Carbs: 6 g Protein: 6 g

Chapter 2:
Dips

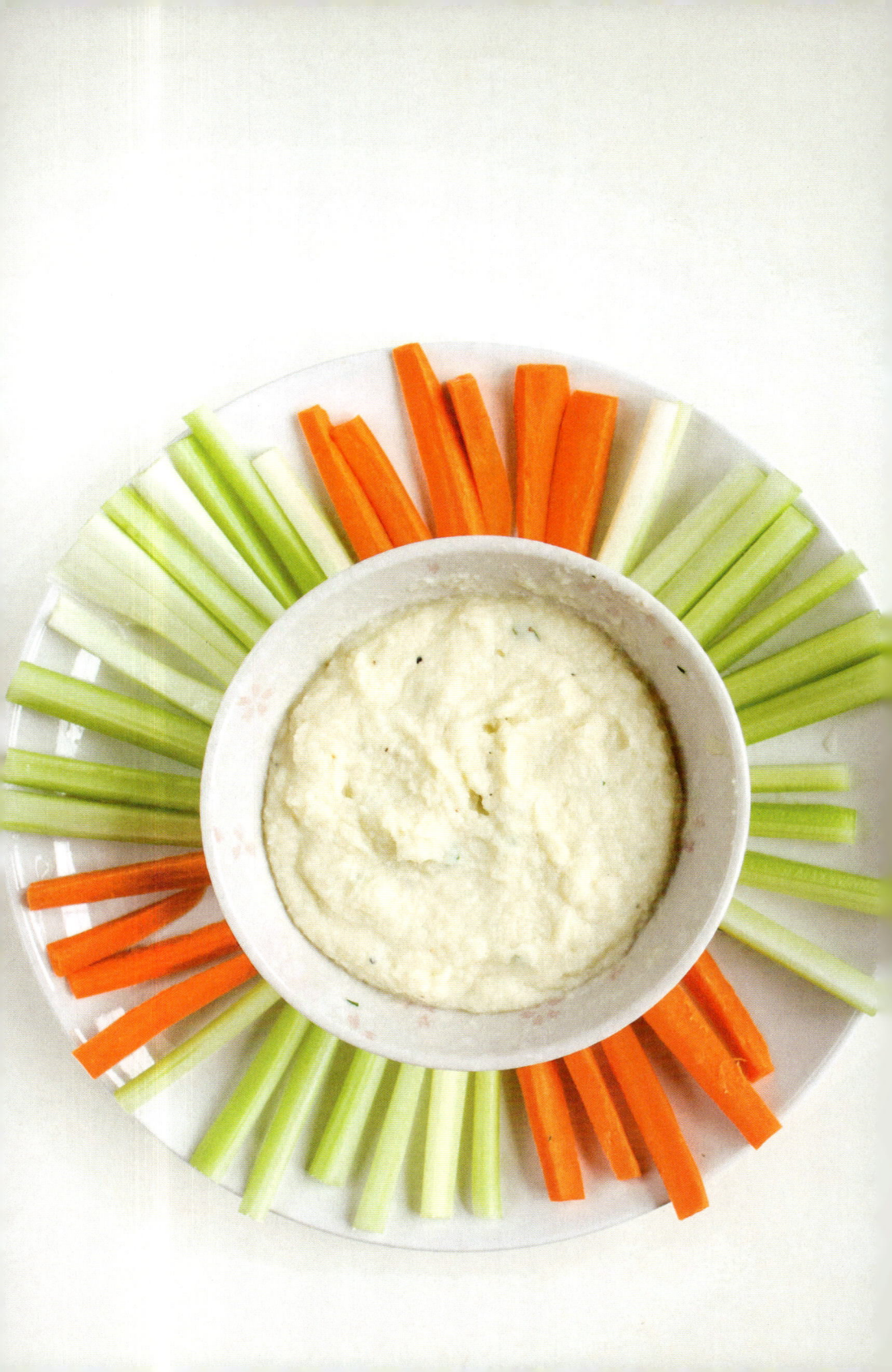

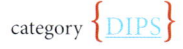
"Hummus" with Cauliflower and Tahini

Prep Time: 10 minutes
Cook Time: 10 minutes
Yield: 4 servings

INGREDIENTS

- 1/2 head (approx. 300 g) cauliflower, broken into florets
- 3 Tablespoons (45 ml) mayo
- 3 cloves of garlic, peeled
- 2 Tablespoons (30 ml) lemon juice
- 1 Tablespoon (15 ml) white tahini (sesame seed paste)
- Sea salt and freshly ground black pepper, to taste

INSTRUCTIONS

1. Steam the cauliflower until softened. Drain the water well.
2. Place steamed cauliflower into a blender and blend really well with the rest of the ingredients.

Nutritional Data (estimates) - per serving: Does not include celery or carrot sticks
Calories: 124   Fat: 11 g   Total Carbs: 6 g   Fiber: 2 g   Sugar: 2 g   Net Carbs: 4 g   Protein: 2 g

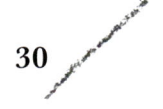

Creamy Garlic Dip

Prep Time: 5 minutes
Cook Time: 0 minutes
Yield: 4 servings

INGREDIENTS

- 10 cloves of garlic, peeled
- 1/4 cup (60 ml) olive oil
- 2 teaspoons (10 ml) lemon juice
- 2 Tablespoons (30 ml) mayo
- Dash of salt

INSTRUCTIONS

1. Blend all the ingredients together well.

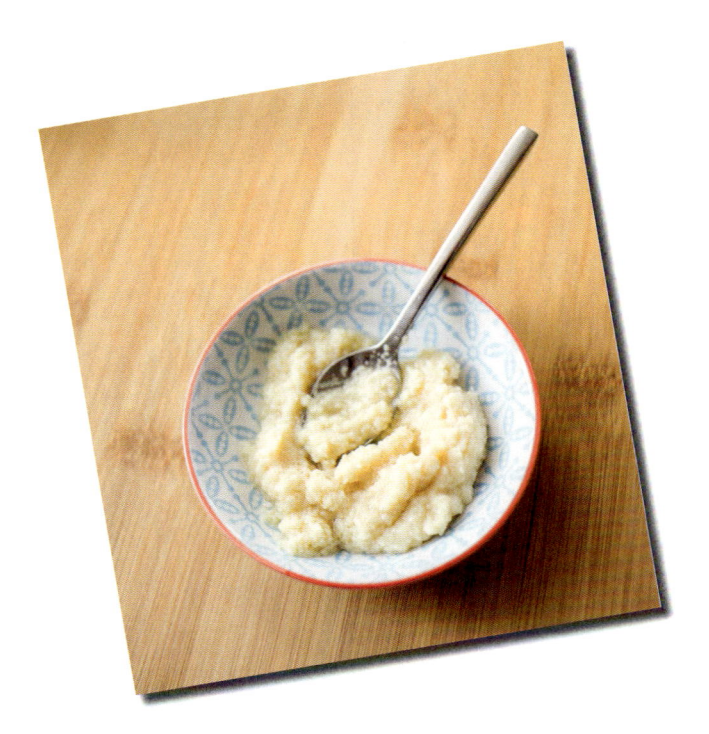

Nutritional Data (estimates) - per serving:
Calories: 179   Fat: 20 g   Total Carbs: 3 g   Fiber: 0 g   Sugar: 0 g   Net Carbs: 3 g   Protein: 0 g

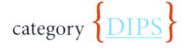
Guacamole

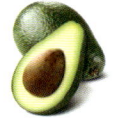

Prep Time: 10 minutes
Cook Time: 0 minutes
Yield: 2 servings

INGREDIENTS

- 1 medium ripe avocado, stone removed
- 1/2 teaspoon (3 ml) lime juice
- 1/2 teaspoon (1 g) onion powder
- 1/2 teaspoon (2 g) garlic powder
- Chili powder, to taste (if you want it spicy)
- 2 cherry tomatoes, finely chopped
- 1 Tablespoon (2 g) cilantro chopped (or 1 teaspoon (1 g) dried cilantro)
- Salt, to taste

INSTRUCTIONS

1. Mash the avocado in a bowl and add in the lime juice.
2. Add in the onion powder, garlic powder, chili powder (optional), cilantro, and diced cherry tomatoes and mix well.
3. Add salt to taste and serve.

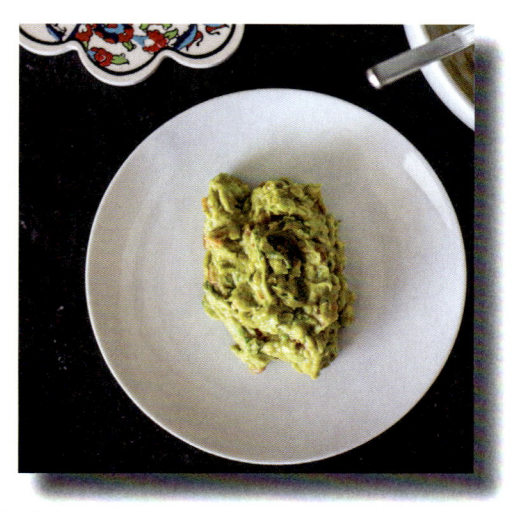

Nutritional Data (estimates) - per serving:
Calories: 300   Fat: 25 g   Total Carbs: 19 g   Fiber: 14 g   Sugar: 3 g   Net Carbs: 5 g   Protein: 4 g

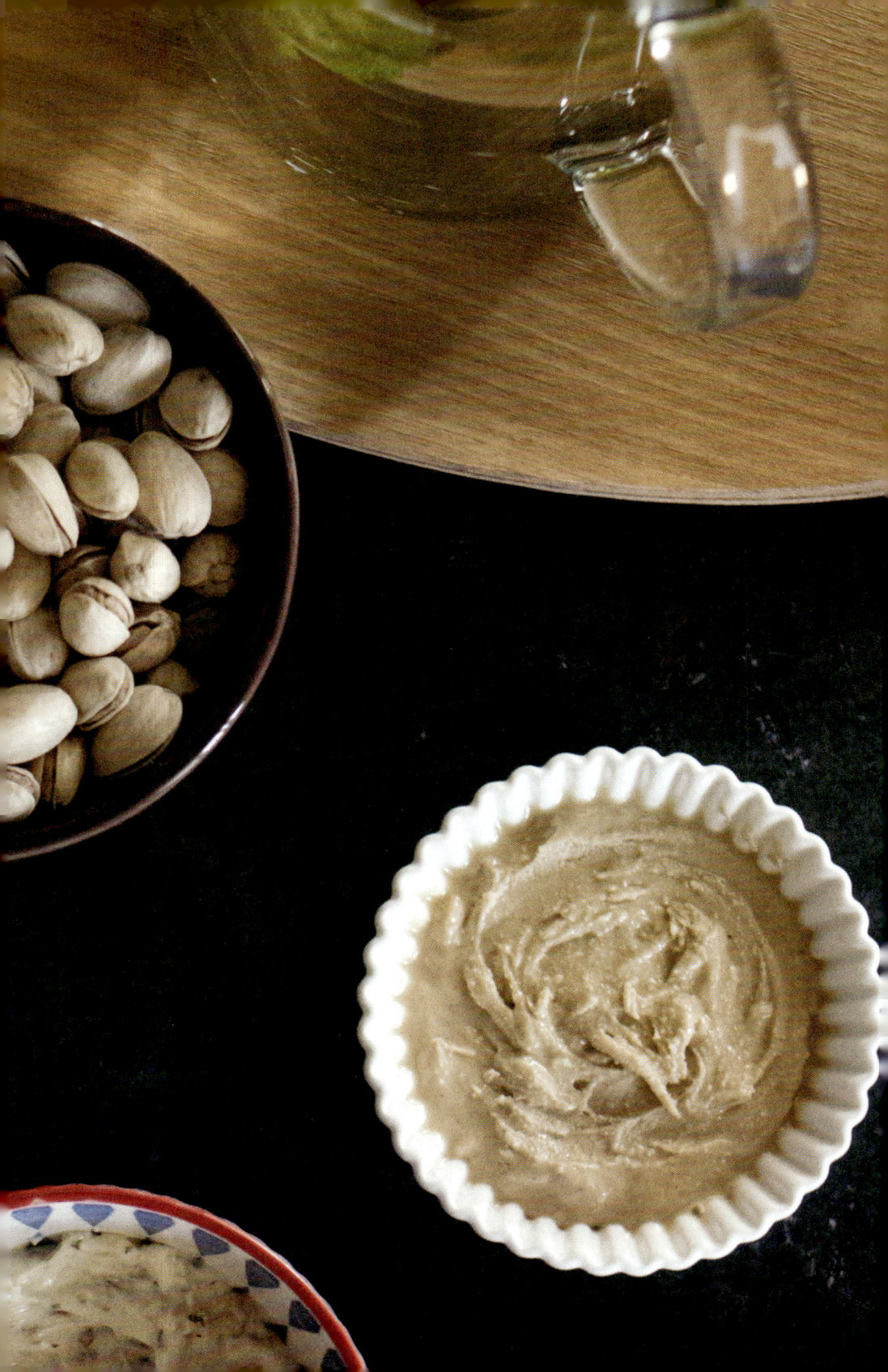

category {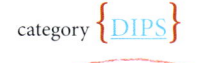DIPS}

Hawaiian "Hummus"

Prep Time: 5 minutes
Cook Time: 0 minutes
Yield: 4 servings

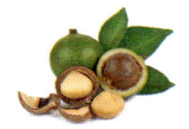

INGREDIENTS

- 1 cup (128 g) macadamia nuts
- 3 Tablespoons (45 ml) lemon juice
- 3 cloves of garlic, peeled
- 2 Tablespoons (30 ml) avocado oil, to get it blending (add more if needed)
- Salt and pepper, to taste

INSTRUCTIONS

1. Place all ingredients into a food processor or blender and blend until smooth.

Nutritional Data (estimates) - per serving:
Calories: 306 Fat: 31 g Total Carbs: 6 g Fiber: 4 g Sugar: 1 g Net Carbs: 2 g Protein: 3 g

Roasted Cauliflower Dip

Prep Time: 10 minutes
Cook Time: 30 minutes
Yield: 2 servings

INGREDIENTS

- 1/2 head (approx. 300 g) cauliflower, broken into florets
- 3 Tablespoons (45 ml) olive oil, divided
- 3 cloves of garlic, peeled
- 2 Tablespoons (30 ml) lemon juice
- 2 teaspoons (10 ml) almond butter
- Sea salt and freshly ground black pepper, to taste
- 1 teaspoon (2 g) fresh parsley, finely chopped
- Cherry tomatoes and cucumber batons, to serve with

INSTRUCTIONS

1. Preheat oven to 400 F (200 C).
2. Toss the cauliflower florets in 2 tablespoons of olive oil.
3. Spread the cauliflower florets out on a greased baking tray. Take the garlic cloves as they are and secure inside a small foil parcel where no air can escape. Place onto the same tray. Roast both the garlic and cauliflower in the oven for 30 minutes, tossing the cauliflower after 15 minutes to ensure even roasting.
4. Remove the roasted cauliflower from the oven (which should have completely softened) and unwrap the garlic. Place both into a mini food processor. Add the lemon juice (check for pips), the almond butter, and the additional tablespoon of olive oil and blend the mixture to a smooth puree.
5. Season with salt and pepper to your liking. Top with parsley and serve with cherry tomatoes and cucumber batons, or any other vegetables that your daily macros will allow.

Nutritional Data (estimates) - per serving:
Calories: 249   Fat: 24 g   Total Carbs: 10 g   Fiber: 4 g   Sugar: 4 g   Net Carbs: 6 g   Protein: 4 g

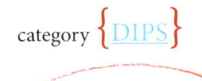

Roasted Eggplant Dip

Prep Time: 10 minutes
Cook Time: 40 minutes
Yield: 6 servings

INGREDIENTS

- 1 large eggplant (approx. 1 lb or 450 g)
- 4 cloves of garlic, peeled
- 2 Tablespoons (30 ml) fresh lemon juice
- 1 Tablespoon (15 ml) coconut cream (from the top of refrigerated cans of coconut milk)
- 1 Tablespoon (15 ml) tahini paste
- Salt and pepper, to taste
- 1 teaspoon (3 g) sesame seeds, for garnish

INSTRUCTIONS

1. Preheat oven to 400 F (200 C).

2. Prick the eggplant a few times with a fork. Then place on a baking tray and roast for 30-40 minutes until tender.

3. If you want a smoky flavor, then place the eggplant under the broiler for a few minutes to blacken the skin a bit.

4. Let the eggplant cool, then cut in half and scoop out the flesh.

5. Blend the eggplant flesh with the garlic, lemon juice, coconut cream, tahini paste, salt and pepper. Adjust seasoning to taste.

6. Spoon into a bowl and sprinkle with sesame seeds for garnish.

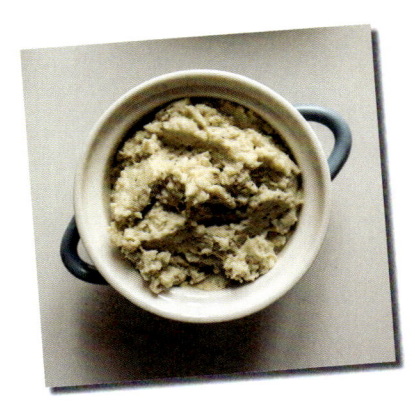

Nutritional Data (estimates) - per serving:
Calories: 45 Fat: 2 g Total Carbs: 6 g Fiber: 3 g Sugar: 2 g Net Carbs: 3 g Protein: 1 g

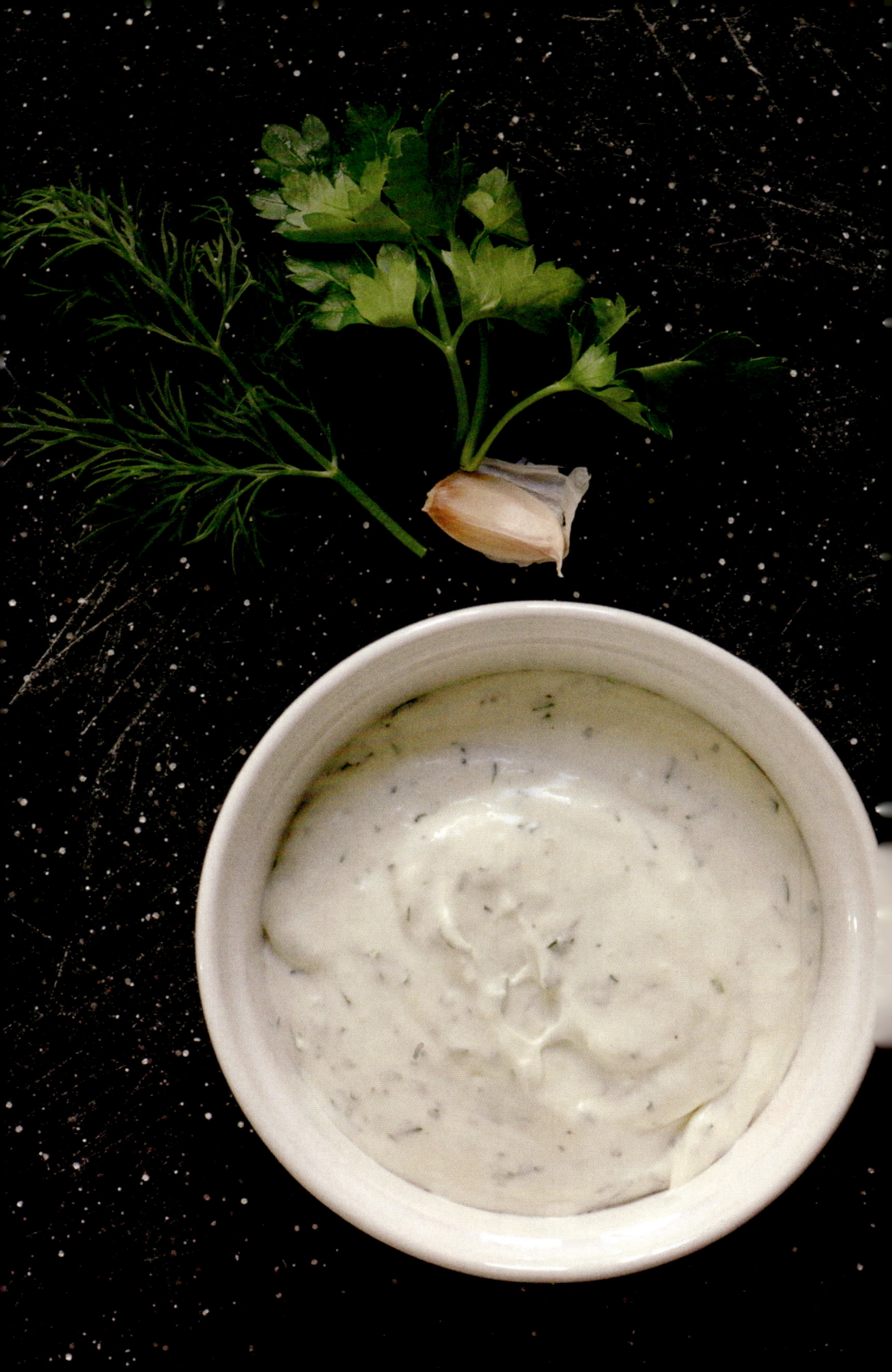

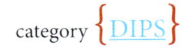

Herb Ranch Dip

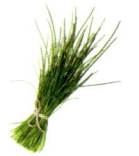

Prep Time: 5 minutes
Cook Time: 0 minutes
Yield: 4 servings

INGREDIENTS

- 1/4 cup (60 ml) mayo
- 1/4 cup (60 ml) coconut cream (from the top of refrigerated cans of coconut milk)
- 1 teaspoon (5 ml) lemon juice
- 1 clove of garlic, peeled and finely diced
- 1/2 teaspoon (1 g) onion powder
- 1 Tablespoon (2 g) fresh parsley, finely chopped (or 1 teaspoon dried parsley)
- 1 Tablespoon (2 g) fresh chives, finely chopped (or omit)
- 1 teaspoon (1 g) fresh dill, finely chopped (or 1/2 teaspoon (0.5 g) dried dill)
- Dash of salt
- Dash of pepper

INSTRUCTIONS

1. Mix together the mayo, coconut cream, lemon juice, onion powder, salt, and pepper with a fork.
2. Gently fold in the finely diced garlic and fresh herbs.

Nutritional Data (estimates) - per serving:
Calories: 131   Fat: 15 g   Total Carbs: 1 g   Fiber: 0 g   Sugar: 0 g   Net Carbs: 1 g   Protein: 0 g

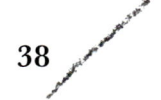

Buffalo Chicken Dip

Prep Time: 10 minutes
Cook Time: 30 minutes
Yield: 8 servings

INGREDIENTS

- 2 chicken breasts (approx. 1 lb or 450 g), diced and sauteed in coconut oil (or 3 cups of cooked chicken meat)
- 1 cup (240 ml) mayo
- 1/3 cup (80 ml) hot sauce (adjust if you don't want it as spicy)
- 2 Tablespoons (30 ml) mustard
- 1 Tablespoon (7 g) onion powder
- 1 Tablespoon (10 g) garlic powder
- Salt and pepper, to taste

INSTRUCTIONS

1. Preheat oven to 350 F (175 C).

2. Shred the cooked chicken and mix with the rest of the ingredients. (Cook the chicken first if you don't have cooked chicken available.)

3. Pour the mixture into a small casserole dish (or 8-by-8 inch pan) and bake for 25-30 minutes until bubbling.

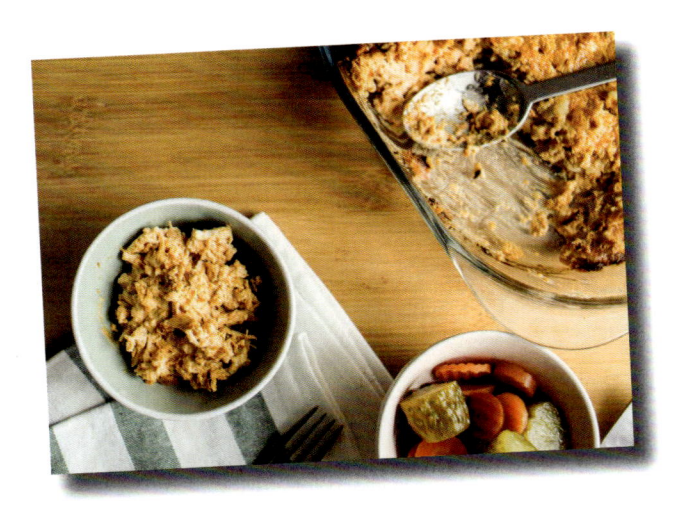

Nutritional Data (estimates) - per serving:
Calories: 404   Fat: 39 g   Total Carbs: 2 g   Fiber: 0 g   Sugar: 1 g   Net Carbs: 2 g   Protein: 16 g

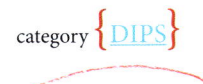

Faux French Onion Dip

Prep Time: 10 minutes
Cook Time: 5 minutes
Yield: 4 servings

INGREDIENTS

- 1/2 onion, diced
- 2 Tablespoons (30 ml) avocado oil,
to cook onions with
- 1/2 cup (120 ml) mayo
- 1 Tablespoon (10 g) garlic powder or
2 cloves of garlic, finely chopped
- 1 Tablespoon (7 g) dried onion flakes
- 1 Tablespoon (3 g) dried parsley
- Salt and pepper, to taste

INSTRUCTIONS

1. Heat the avocado oil in a hot frying pan. Add the diced onion to the pan and fry until slightly browned.

2. Place the onions on a plate and let cool for 5 minutes.

3. Mix everything together and season with salt and pepper, to taste.

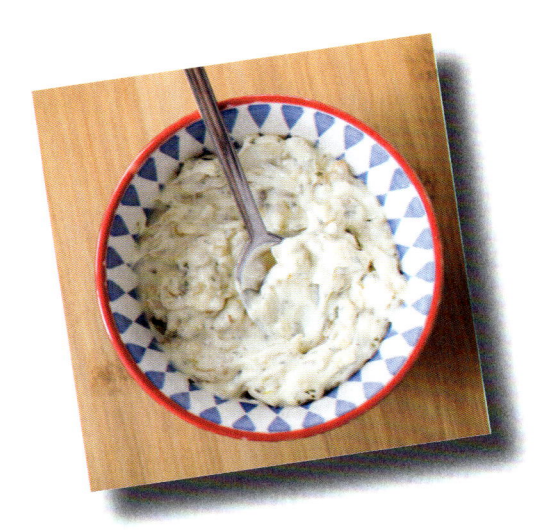

Nutritional Data (estimates) - per serving:
Calories: 278   Fat: 31 g   Total Carbs: 4 g   Fiber: 1 g   Sugar: 2 g   Net Carbs: 3 g   Protein: 0 g

Chapter 3:
Baked Goods

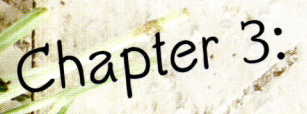

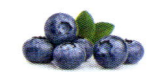

Blueberry Muffins

Prep Time: 10 minutes
Cook Time: 20 minutes
Yield: 6 muffins

INGREDIENTS

- 1.5 cups (180 g) almond flour
- 1/4 cup (60 ml) ghee, melted but not too hot
- 2 eggs, whisked
- 1 Tablespoon (15 ml) vanilla extract
- Erythritol or stevia, to taste
- 1/2 teaspoon (4 g) baking soda
- Dash of salt
- Approx. 24 blueberries (1/2 cup), divided

INSTRUCTIONS

1. Preheat oven to 350 F (175 C).

2. Melt the ghee in a mixing bowl. Add in the almond flour, eggs, vanilla extract, sweetener, baking soda, and salt. Mix everything together well.

3. Break up the blueberries gently by poking with a sharp knife to burst the skin. Stir half of the blueberries into the mixture.

4. Save 12 blueberries to put on top near the end.

5. Line a muffin pan with muffin liners or grease it. Spoon the mixture into the muffin pan (to around 3/4 full). Makes 6 muffins. Place 2 blueberries at the top of each muffin.

6. Bake for 18-20 minutes until a toothpick comes out clean when you insert it into a muffin.

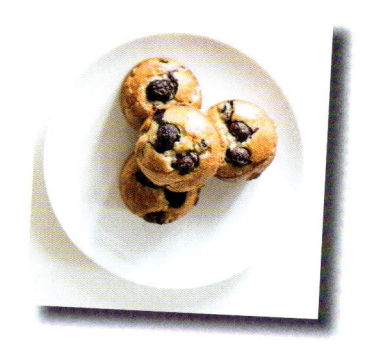

Nutritional Data (estimates) - per muffin:
Calories: 240   Fat: 22 g   Total Carbs: 6 g   Fiber: 3 g   Sugar: 2 g   Net Carbs: 3 g   Protein: 7 g

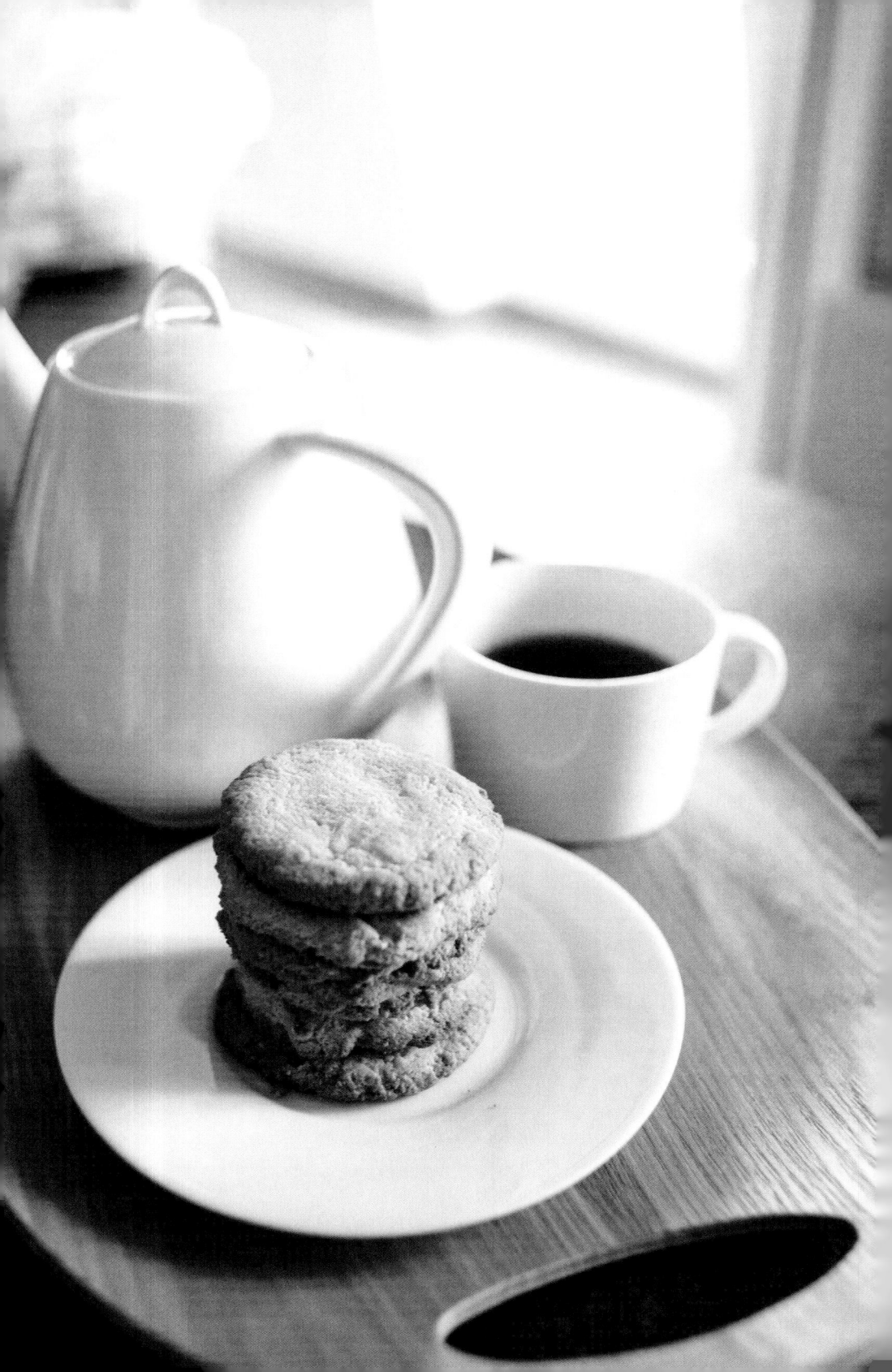

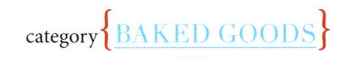
Almond Flour Cookies with Lemon Zest

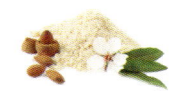

Prep Time: 10 minutes
Cooking Time: 20 minutes
Yield: 4 servings

INGREDIENTS

- 1 cup (120 g) almond flour
- 1 egg, whisked
- 3 Tablespoons (45 ml) ghee, melted
- Erythritol or stevia, to taste
- 1 teaspoon (5 ml) vanilla extract
- 1 Tablespoon lemon zest
- 1/2 teaspoon (2 ml) lemon extract
- Pinch of (1 g) baking soda

INSTRUCTIONS

1. Preheat oven to 350 F (175 C).

2. Mix all the ingredients together in a mixing bowl to form a dough.

3. Chill the dough for 20 minutes in the fridge.

4. Using a stencil or cookie cutter, or just your hands, form the dough into 8 small round cookies.

5. Place on a parchment paper-lined baking tray.

6. Bake for 15-20 minutes until the cookies are slightly browned.

7. Remove from oven and place on a cooling rack. They'll crisp up after cooling.

Nutritional Data (estimates) - per serving:
Calories: 242   Fat: 23 g   Total Carbs: 5 g   Fiber: 3 g   Sugar: 1 g   Net Carbs: 2 g   Protein: 7 g

"Cornbread" Muffins

Prep Time: 10 minutes
Cook Time: 20 minutes
Yield: 6 muffins

INGREDIENTS

- 3/4 cup (90 g) almond flour
- 1/4 cup (30 g) coconut flour
- 2 teaspoons (9 g) baking powder
- 1 teaspoon (5 g) salt
- 2 Tablespoons (30 ml) ghee, melted but not too hot
- 3 eggs, whisked
- 1/2 cup (120 ml) coconut milk
- 1 Tablespoon (12 g) erythritol or stevia, to taste

INSTRUCTIONS

1. Preheat oven to 350 F (175 C).

2. Grease muffin pan or use muffin liners or silicone muffin pan.

3. Mix together all ingredients well in a large bowl.

4. Pour the batter into the muffin pan (makes 6 muffins).

6. Bake for 18-20 minutes until a toothpick comes out clean when you insert it into a muffin.

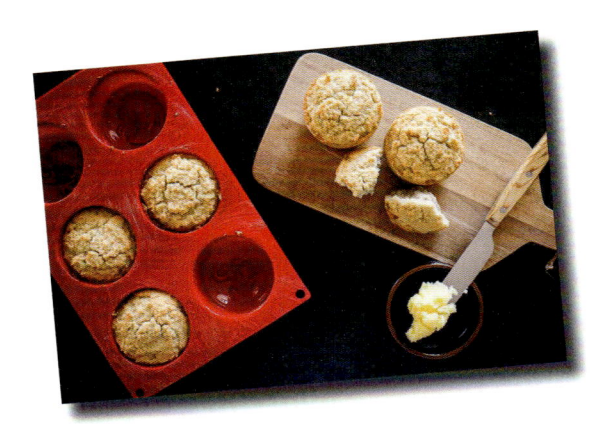

Nutritional Data (estimates) - per muffin:
Calories: 191   Fat: 17 g   Total Carbs: 5 g   Fiber: 3 g   Sugar: 1 g   Net Carbs: 2 g   Protein: 6 g

Ginger Coconut Cookies

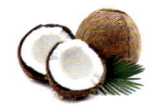

Prep Time: 10 minutes
Cook Time: 20 minutes
Yield: 4 servings

INGREDIENTS

- 2/3 cup (80 g) almond meal
- 1/4 cup (28 g) coconut flour
- 2 Tablespoons (10 g) coconut flakes
- 1 egg, whisked
- 3 Tablespoons (45 ml) ghee, melted
- Erythritol or stevia, to taste
- 1 teaspoon (5 ml) vanilla extract
- 2 teaspoons (4 g) ginger powder
- Pinch of (1 g) baking soda

INSTRUCTIONS

1. Preheat oven to 350 F (175 C).

2. Combine all the ingredients in a mixing bowl to form a dough.

3. If you have time, place the dough in the fridge for 15-20 minutes to chill.

4. Then using a cookie cutter, form small cookies (approx. 8 cookies).

5. Place on a baking tray and bake for 15-20 minutes until they are just slightly browned on top.

6. Remove from oven and place on a cooling rack.

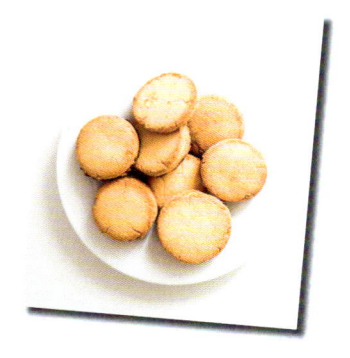

Nutritional Data (estimates) - per serving:
Calories: 237   Fat: 21 g   Total Carbs: 7 g   Fiber: 5 g   Sugar: 1 g   Net Carbs: 2 g   Protein: 6 g

category {BAKED GOODS}

Chocolate Brownies

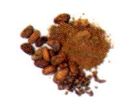

Prep Time: 10 minutes
Cook Time: 15 minutes
Yield: 9 servings

INGREDIENTS

- 6 Tablespoons (90 ml) coconut oil or ghee, melted but not too hot
- 3 eggs, whisked
- 2 teaspoons (10 ml) vanilla extract
- 1 cup (120 g) almond flour
- 1 cup (80 g) unsweetened cacao powder
- 2 Tablespoons (30 ml) coconut cream (from the top of refrigerated cans of coconut milk)
- 1/2 cup (96 g) granulated erythritol or stevia, to taste

INSTRUCTIONS

1. Preheat the oven to 350 F (175 C).

2. Whisk the eggs well, then stir in the vanilla extract, coconut cream and coconut oil (ensuring the coconut oil is not too hot, else it will scramble the eggs). Mix well and set aside.

3. Combine the almond flour, unsweetened cacao powder, and sweetener in a bowl.

4. Add the wet egg mixture to the almond flour mixture and combine until fully incorporated.

5. Tip the mixture into a small, greased baking dish (approx. 8-by-8-inch), smooth down the top and place in the oven for 15 minutes.

6. Use a cake tester to ensure the brownies have cooked, then remove and allow to cool before slicing into 9 squares.

Nutritional Data (estimates) - per serving:
Calories: 210 Fat: 18 g Total Carbs: 8 g Fiber: 5 g Sugar: 1 g Net Carbs: 3 g Protein: 7 g

Raspberry Lemon Muffins

Prep Time: 10 minutes
Cook Time: 20 minutes
Yield: 12 muffins

INGREDIENTS

- 3 cups (360 g) almond flour
- 1/2 cup (120 ml) ghee or coconut oil, melted but not too hot
- 4 eggs, whisked
- 1 cup raspberries (68 g)
- 2 Tablespoons lemon zest
- 1 Tablespoon (15 ml) vanilla extract
- 1/4 cup (48 g) erythritol or stevia, to taste
- 1 teaspoon (4 g) baking soda

INSTRUCTIONS

1. Preheat oven to 350 F (175 C).

2. Mix together all the ingredients in a large mixing bowl.

3. Pour into muffin pans (use silicone muffin pans or grease the metal pans).
Makes 12 muffins.

4. Bake for 18-20 minutes until a toothpick comes out clean when you insert it
into a muffin.

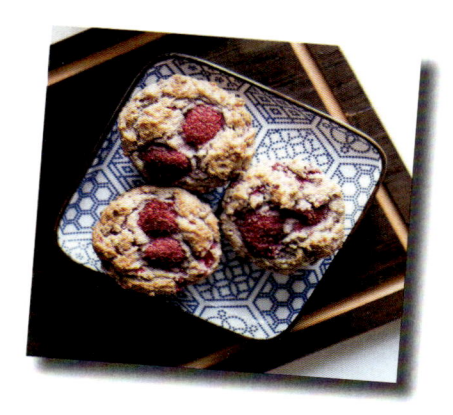

Nutritional Data (estimates) - per serving:
Calories: 258   Fat: 22 g   Total Carbs: 10 g   Fiber: 6 g   Sugar: 3 g   Net Carbs: 4 g   Protein: 7 g

category {BAKED GOODS}

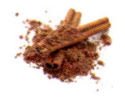

Cinnamon Donut Balls

Prep Time: 10 minutes
Cook Time: 15 minutes
Yield: 6 servings

INGREDIENTS

- 1 cup (120 g) almond flour
- 1/4 cup (48 g) granulated erythritol or stevia, to taste
- 1 egg, whisked
- 2 Tablespoons (30 ml) ghee, melted but not hot
- 1 teaspoon (4 g) baking powder
- 2 Tablespoons (14 g) cinnamon
- 1 teaspoon (2 g) ginger powder

INSTRUCTIONS

1. Preheat oven to 350 F (175 C).
2. Combine all the ingredients together in a mixing bowl.
3. Form 12 balls from the dough.
4. Place on a piece of parchment paper and bake for 15 minutes.

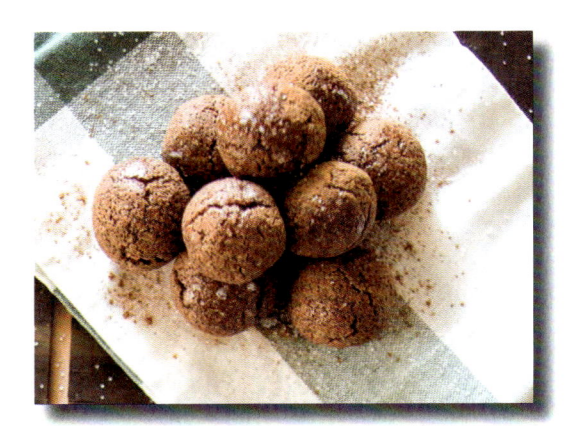

Nutritional Data (estimates) - per serving:
Calories: 148   Fat: 13 g   Total Carbs: 5 g   Fiber: 3 g   Sugar: 1 g   Net Carbs: 2 g   Protein: 4 g

Cinnamon Orange Muffins

Prep Time: 10 minutes
Cook Time: 20 minutes
Yield: 12 muffins

INGREDIENTS

- 3 cups (360 g) almond flour
- 1/2 cup (120 ml) ghee or coconut oil, melted but not too hot
- 4 eggs, whisked
- 3 Tablespoons (18 g) cinnamon
- 1 teaspoon (2 g) nutmeg
- 1/4 teaspoon (1 g) cloves
- 3 Tablespoons orange zest
- 1 teaspoon (5 ml) lemon juice
- 1 teaspoon (4 g) baking soda
- 1/4 cup (48 g) erythritol or stevia, to taste

INSTRUCTIONS

1. Preheat oven to 350 F (175 C).

2. Mix together all the ingredients in a large mixing bowl.

3. Pour batter into muffin pans (use silicone muffin pans or grease the metal muffin pans). This recipe makes 12 muffins.

4. Bake in the preheated oven for 18-20 minutes until a toothpick comes out clean when you insert it into a muffin.

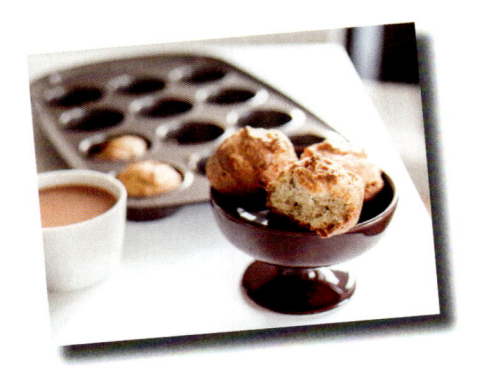

Nutritional Data (estimates) - per serving:
Calories: 243   Fat: 22 g   Total Carbs: 6 g   Fiber: 4 g   Sugar: 1 g   Net Carbs: 2 g   Protein: 7 g

Chapter 4:
Game Night

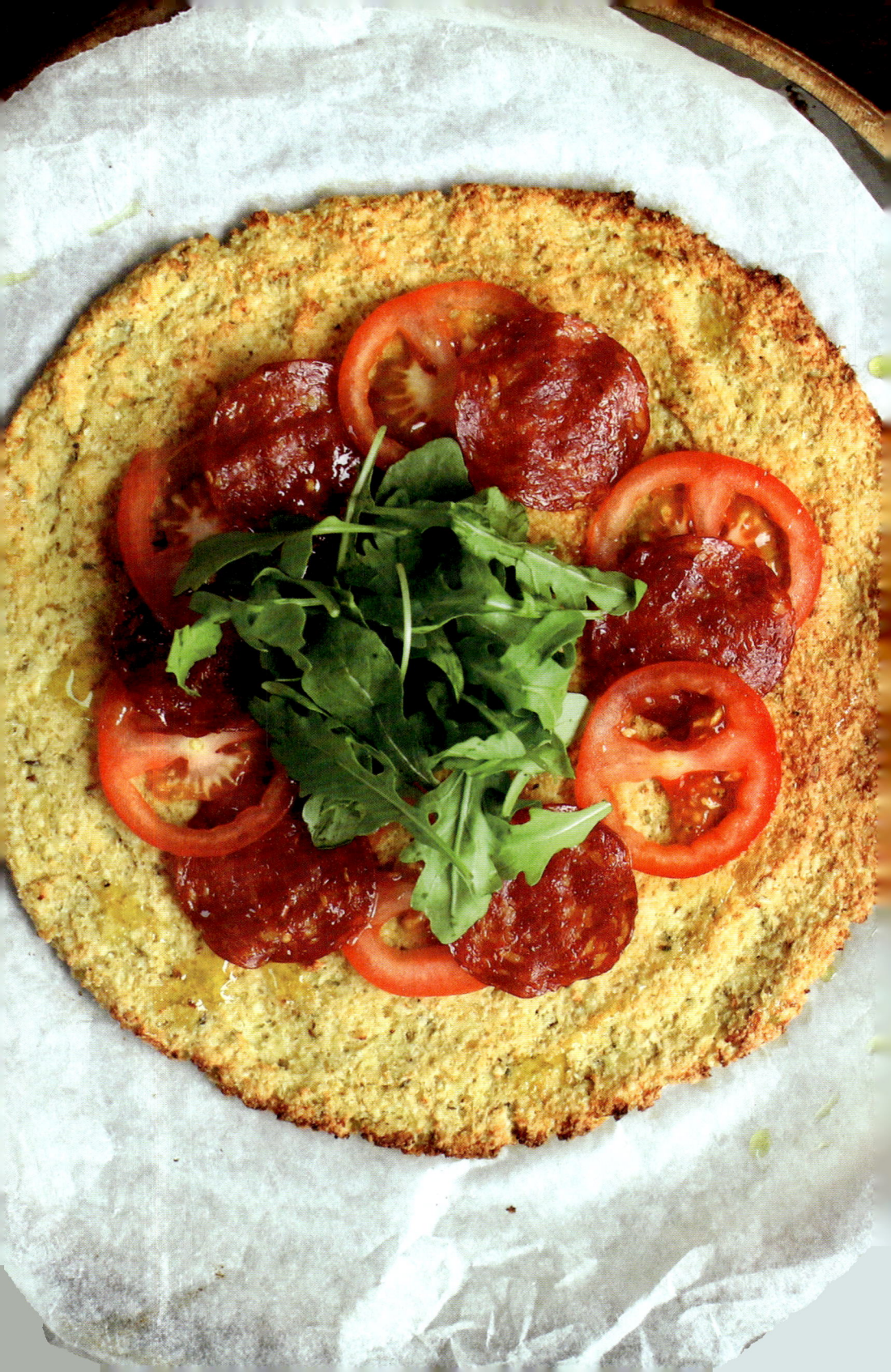

Cauliflower Pizza

Prep Time: 20 minutes
Cook Time: 26 minutes
Yield: 2 servings

INGREDIENTS
- 1/2 head (approx. 300 g) cauliflower, broken into florets
- 2/3 cup (80 g) almond flour
- 1 teaspoon (3 g) garlic powder
- 1 teaspoon (2 g) onion powder
- 1 teaspoon (1 g) dried oregano
- 2 teaspoons (10 ml) olive oil (plus additional for drizzling)
- 1 egg, whisked
- 1 small tomato (90 g), sliced
- 12 slices of pepperoni or other topping of your choice
- 2 oz (56 g) arugula

INSTRUCTIONS
1. Preheat oven to 350 F (175 C).

2. Place cauliflower florets in a microwave-safe bowl. Microwave, partially covered, on high for 5 to 6 minutes. Carefully remove from microwave and pour the cauliflower onto a clean dish towel or muslin. Set aside and let cool. Alternatively, you can roast or steam the cauliflower florets to soften them.

3. Once cool enough to touch, wrap the dish towel or muslin around the cauliflower and squeeze out the excess liquid as much as possible.

4. Blend or food process the cauliflower with the almond flour, garlic powder, onion powder, dried oregano, olive oil, and egg. Remove from food processor and knead until it forms a ball of dough.

5. Place the dough on a parchment paper-lined baking tray and press or roll into a round, thin pizza shape.

6. Place in the oven and bake for 10 minutes. Remove from oven and top with the tomato and pepperoni slices. Return to the oven and bake for an additional 10 minutes.

7. Drizzle the baked pizza with additional olive oil and top with arugula. Slice into the desired amount of pieces and serve immediately.

Nutritional Data (estimates) - per serving:
Calories: 436   Fat: 36 g   Total Carbs: 19 g   Fiber: 8 g   Sugar: 7 g   Net Carbs: 11 g   Protein: 16 g

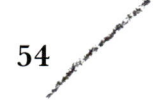

Asian Chicken Wings

Prep Time: 10 minutes
Cook Time: 35 minutes
Yield: 5 servings

INGREDIENTS

- 2 lbs (900 g) chicken wings (approx. 10 wings), with skin on
- 2 Tablespoons (30 ml) sesame oil
- 1/4 cup (60 ml) gluten-free tamari sauce or coconut aminos
- 1 Tablespoon (6 g) ginger powder
- 2 teaspoons (10 ml) white wine vinegar
- 3 cloves of garlic, peeled and minced
- 1 teaspoon (5 g) sea salt

INSTRUCTIONS

1. Preheat oven to 400 F (200 C).
2. In a large container toss the sesame oil, tamari sauce, ginger powder, vinegar, garlic, and salt.
3. Whisk to thoroughly combine all ingredients. Add the chicken wings to the mixture.
4. Place the wings (meaty side up) on a parchment paper-lined baking sheet.
5. Bake for 30-35 minutes until the skin is crispy. (Drizzle leftover marinade on the wings halfway through.)
6. Turn on the broiler for a few minutes if you want the wings crispier.

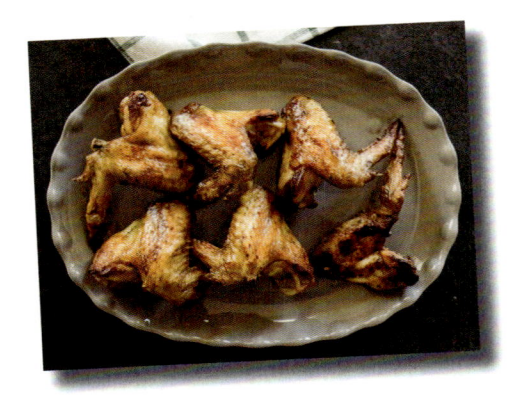

Nutritional Data (estimates) - per serving:
Calories: 277   Fat: 22 g   Total Carbs: 1 g   Fiber: 0 g   Sugar: 0 g   Net Carbs: 1 g   Protein: 18 g

Jalapeño Muffins

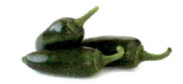

Prep Time: 10 minutes
Cook Time: 20 minutes
Yield: 12 muffins

INGREDIENTS

- 3/4 cup (90 g) almond flour
- 1/4 cup (30 g) coconut flour
- 2 teaspoons (8 g) baking powder
- Dash of salt
- Small amount of stevia or erythritol
- 2 Tablespoons (30 ml) ghee or coconut oil, melted but not hot
- 3 eggs, whisked
- 3/4 cup (180 ml) coconut milk
- 4 jalapeño peppers (56 g), deseeded and finely diced

INSTRUCTIONS

1. Preheat oven to 350 F (175 C).

2. Place all the dry ingredients into a large mixing bowl and mix together.

3. Then add in the ghee or coconut oil, whisked eggs, and coconut milk.

4. Lastly, carefully stir in the chopped jalapeño pepper pieces.

5. Pour the mixture into a greased muffin tray or use muffin liners (makes 12 muffins).

6. Bake for 18-20 minutes until a toothpick inserted into the middle of a muffin comes out clean.

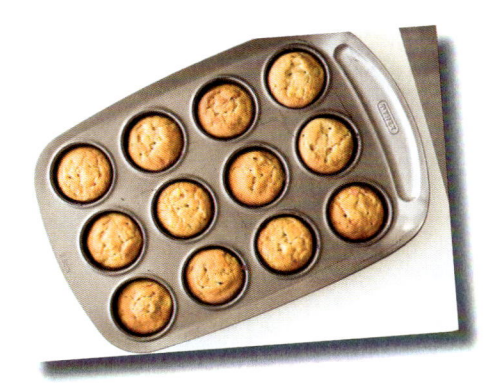

Nutritional Data (estimates) - per muffin:
Calories: 96   Fat: 8 g   Total Carbs: 2 g   Fiber: 2 g   Sugar: 1 g   Net Carbs: 0 g   Protein: 3 g

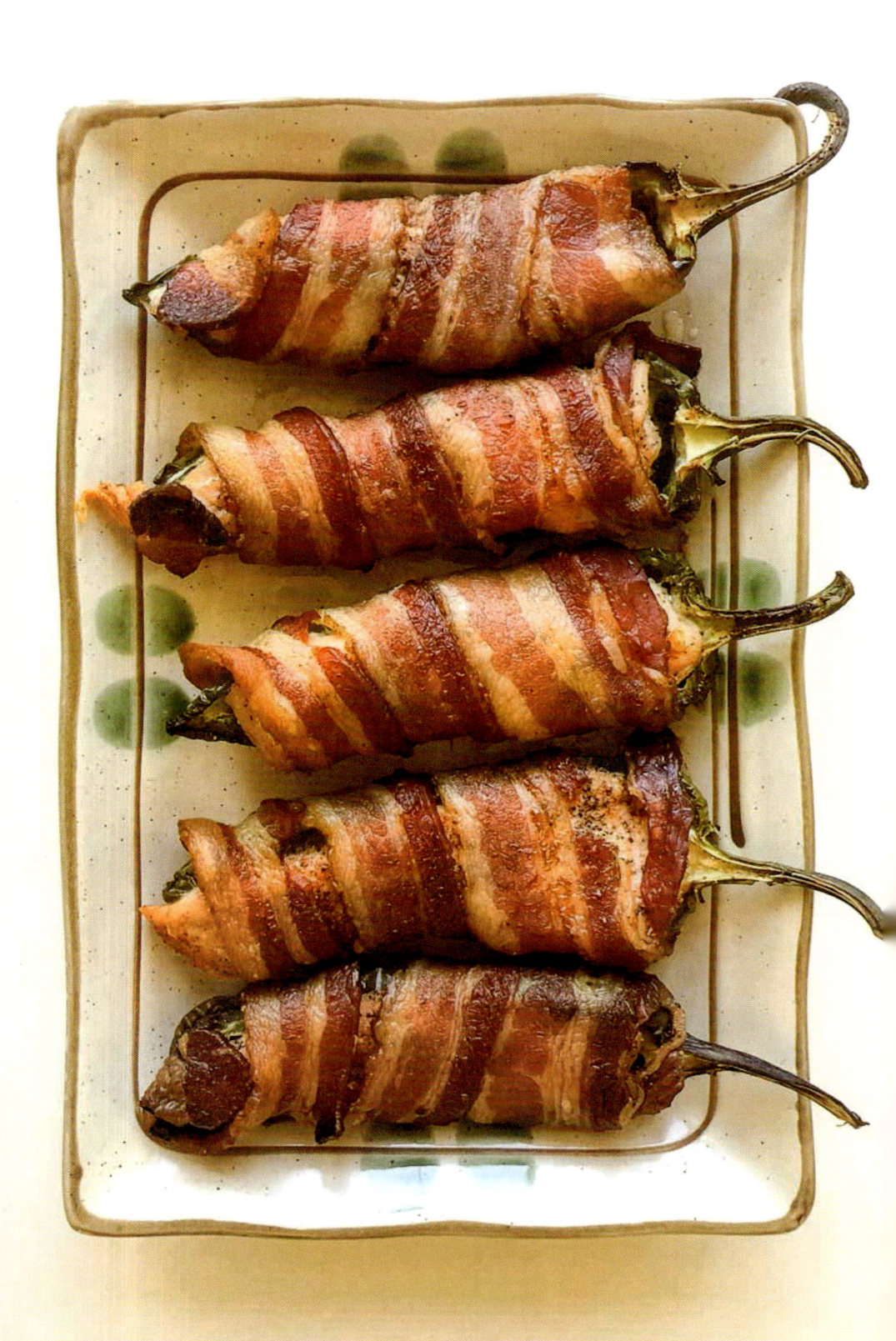

Bacon & Chicken Jalapeño Poppers

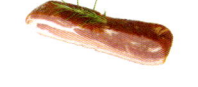

Prep Time: 10 minutes
Cook Time: 50 minutes
Yield: 3 servings

INGREDIENTS

- 1 chicken breast (1/2 lb or 225 g), cut into 6 strips
- 6 slices of bacon, raw
- 3 jalapeño peppers, ribs and seeds removed and sliced in half

INSTRUCTIONS

1. Preheat oven to 350 F (175 C).

2. Line a baking tray with parchment paper.

3. Place one jalapeño half onto a strip of chicken and wrap both together with a slice of bacon. Place, with the bacon ends folded down, onto the lined baking tray.

4. Repeat with remaining chicken, peppers, and bacon.

5. Bake for around 50 minutes. Check the chicken is cooked through and bacon is slightly crispy.

Nutritional Data (estimates) - per serving:
Calories: 389   Fat: 33 g   Total Carbs: 1 g   Fiber: 0 g   Sugar: 0 g   Net Carbs: 1 g   Protein: 22 g

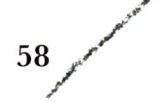

Bacon Wrapped Asparagus

Prep Time: 10 minutes
Cook Time: 30 minutes
Yield: 4 servings

INGREDIENTS

- 16 slices of bacon, raw
- 16 spears of asparagus

INSTRUCTIONS

1. Preheat oven to 400 F (200 C).

2. Wrap each slice of bacon tightly around each asparagus spear.

3. Place on a baking tray and bake for 15 minutes.

4. Use tongs to turn the pieces around and bake for another 10-15 minutes until the bacon starts to get crispy.

5. If the bacon isn't crispy enough to your liking then turn the broiler on and crisp up the bacon for a few minutes.

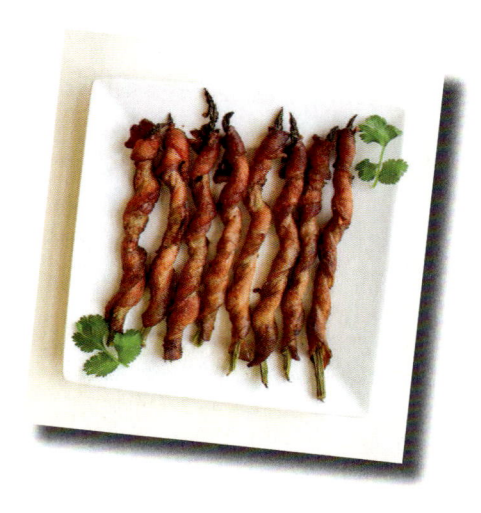

Nutritional Data (estimates) - per serving:
Calories: 524   Fat: 52 g   Total Carbs: 4 g   Fiber: 2 g   Sugar: 2 g   Net Carbs: 2 g   Protein: 12 g

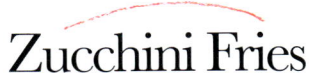
Zucchini Fries

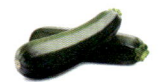

Prep Time: 10 minutes
Cook Time: 30 minutes
Yield: 6 servings

INGREDIENTS

- 5 zucchinis
- 1 cup (112 g) coconut flour
- 2 Tablespoons (14 g) onion powder
- 2 Tablespoons (20 g) garlic powder
- 2 teaspoons (4 g) paprika
- 2 teaspoons (4 g) chili powder
- 1 teaspoon (5 g) salt
- Black pepper, to taste

INSTRUCTIONS

1. Preheat oven to 400 F (200 C).

2. Cut zucchini ensuring the inner fleshy parts are mostly removed and discarded. Then slice the zucchini into 1/4-inch sticks.

3. Combine the coconut flour, onion powder, garlic powder, paprika, chili powder, salt, and freshly ground black pepper in a large bowl. Add the zucchini sticks to the bowl and toss to coat evenly.

4. Spread the sticks evenly on a greased baking tray and cook in the oven for 20 minutes.

5. Shake the tray and cook for an additional 5-10 minutes until golden.

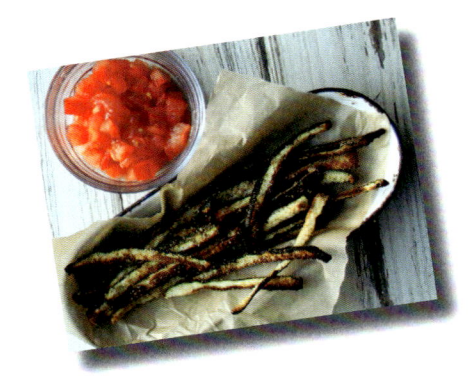

Nutritional Data (estimates) - per serving:
Calories: 101   Fat: 2 g   Total Carbs: 15 g   Fiber: 8 g   Sugar: 5 g   Net Carbs: 7 g   Protein: 4 g

Chapter 5:
Easy Bites

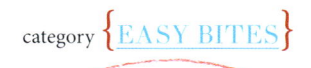

Spicy Roast Beef Salsa Roll-ups

Prep Time: 5 minutes
Cook Time: 0 minutes
Yield: 8 servings

INGREDIENTS
- 8 slices of deli roast beef (or use deli ham or turkey or smoked salmon slices)
- 1 avocado (approx. 1/2 lb or 225 g), stone removed and flesh mashed

For the salsa:
- 1 small tomato, finely diced
- 1/2 small red onion, finely diced
- 1 chili pepper, deseeded and finely chopped (optional)
- Zest and juice of 1/2 lime
- 1 Tablespoon (15 ml) olive oil
- Salt and pepper, to taste

INSTRUCTIONS
1. Make the salsa by tossing all the salsa ingredients together. Drain well.
2. Spread mashed avocado on each roast beef slice. And then spoon some salsa on top and roll up.

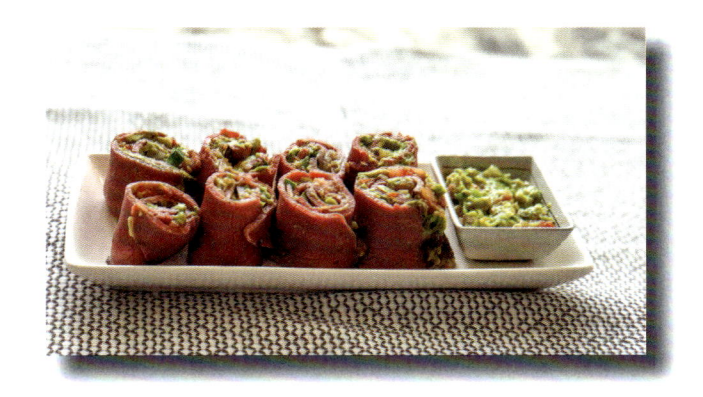

Nutritional Data (estimates) - per serving:
Calories: 88   Fat: 6 g   Total Carbs: 3 g   Fiber: 2 g   Sugar: 1 g   Net Carbs: 1 g   Protein: 6 g

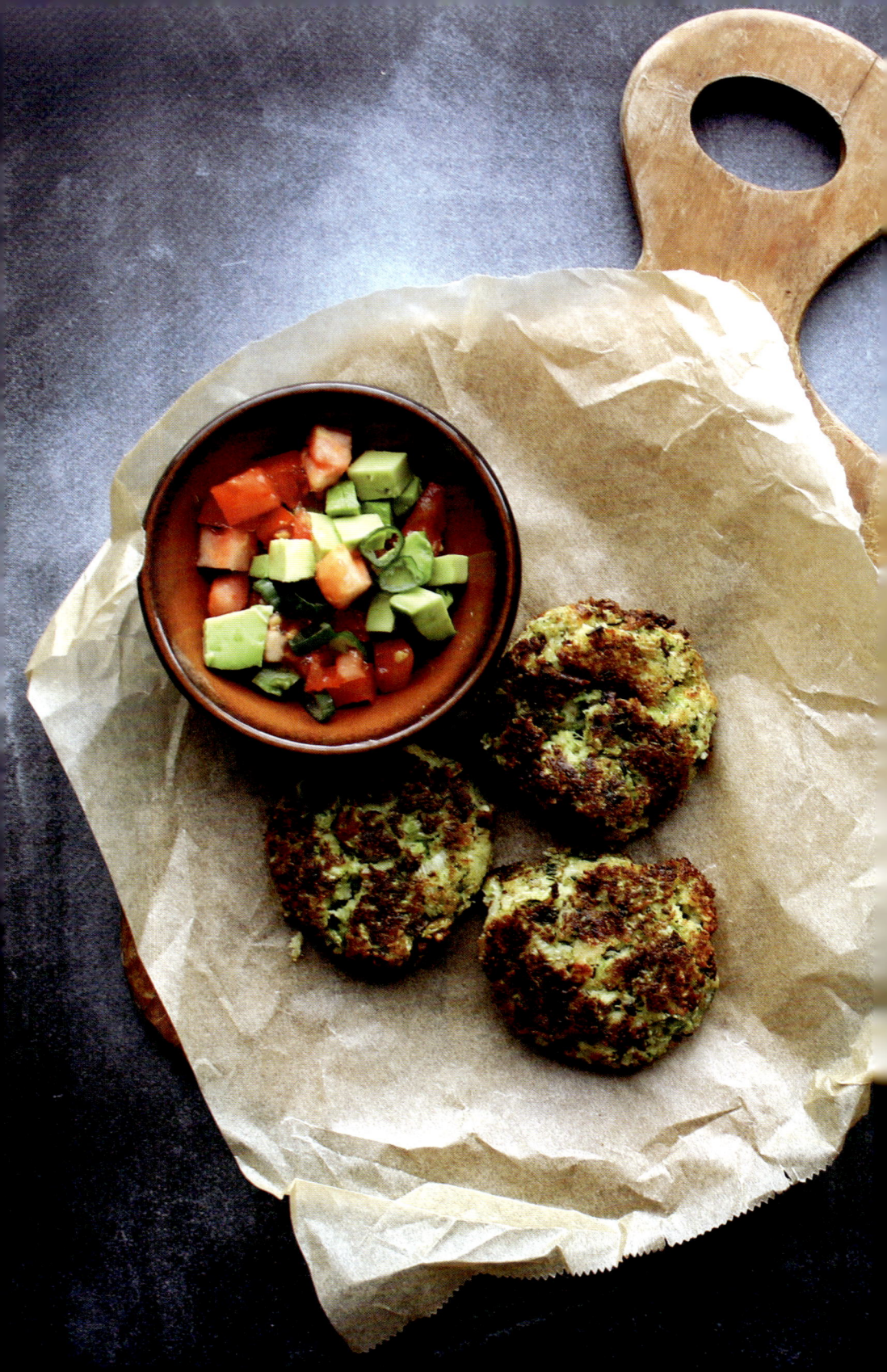

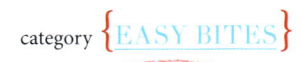

Zucchini Fritters

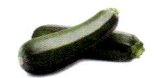

Prep Time: 10 minutes
Cook Time: 20 minutes
Yield: 2 servings

INGREDIENTS

- 4 zucchinis, grated
- 2 green onions (10 g), diced
- 2 Tablespoons (14 g) onion powder
- 2 Tablespoons (20 g) garlic powder
- 2 teaspoons (2 g) dried oregano
- 3/4 cup (84 g) coconut flour
- 2 eggs, whisked
- 1/4 cup (60 ml) olive oil or avocado oil, to cook with
- Salt and freshly ground black pepper, to taste

INSTRUCTIONS

1. Preheat the oven to 350 F (175 C).

2. After grating or food processing the zucchini, squeeze out as much moisture as you can by wrapping it in muslin and squeezing as hard as you can. Squeeze until you have a dry pulp.

3. Combine all the ingredients except the olive oil. Form into 12 balls of approximately 1 oz (30 g) each. Then press into flat patties.

4. Heat the olive oil in a frying pan and carefully place the fritters into the hot oil. Once the bottom is golden and crispy turn them over and cook for a few more minutes until that side is also browned.

5. Then, transfer the fritters to a greased baking tray and bake in oven for 10-15 minutes until fully cooked.

Nutritional Data (estimates) - per serving:
Calories: 181   Fat: 12 g   Total Carbs: 12 g   Fiber: 6 g   Sugar: 4 g   Net Carbs: 6 g   Protein: 5 g

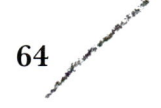

Curry Candied Bacon

Prep Time: 5 minutes
Cook Time: 20 minutes
Yield: 4 servings

INGREDIENTS

- 8 slices of bacon, raw
- 2 Tablespoons (24 g) erythritol
- 1 Tablespoon (7 g) curry powder

INSTRUCTIONS

1. Preheat oven to 400 F (200 C).

2. Lay the bacon slices on a baking rack.

3. Mix the curry powder with the erythritol and rub over the bacon slices.

4. Bake the bacon until crispy (approx. 20 minutes).

5. Enjoy as entire slices or crumble into small pieces for a snack.

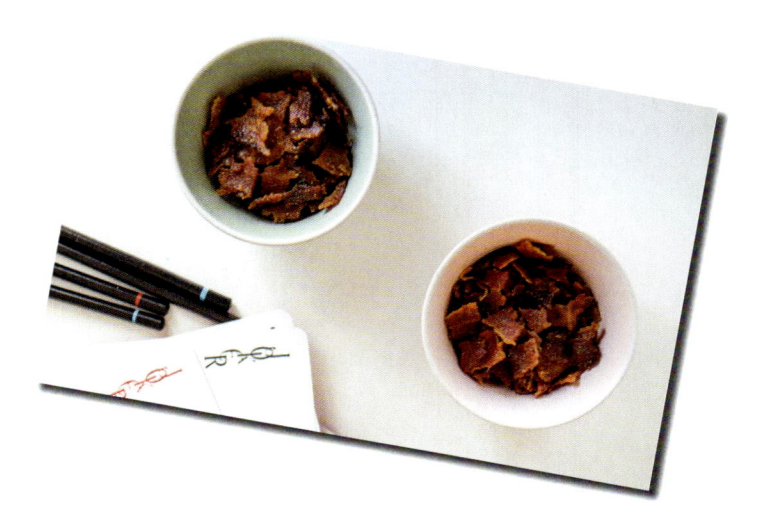

Nutritional Data (estimates) - per serving:
Calories: 261   Fat: 26 g   Total Carbs: 1 g   Fiber: 1 g   Sugar: 0 g   Net Carbs: 0 g   Protein: 6 g

Buffalo Cauliflower Bites

Prep Time: 10 minutes
Cook Time: 25 minutes
Yield: 4 servings

INGREDIENTS

- 1 head (approx. 1.5 lb or 600 g) cauliflower, broken into small florets
- 3 Tablespoons (45 ml) avocado oil
- 2 teaspoons (7 g) garlic powder
- 1 teaspoon salt (5 g) or to taste
- 2 Tablespoons (30 ml) ghee, melted
- 1/4 cup (60 ml) hot sauce

INSTRUCTIONS

1. Preheat oven to 450 F (230 C).

2. In a large mixing bowl, combine the avocado oil, garlic powder, and salt.

3. Toss the cauliflower florets in the mixture.

4. Place the cauliflower florets on a baking sheet and bake for 15 minutes.

5. Meanwhile, melt the ghee and combine with the hot sauce.

6. Toss the cauliflower florets in the hot sauce mixture and bake for another 5-10 minutes until slightly browned.

7. Serve with the herb ranch dip (see recipe on page 37).

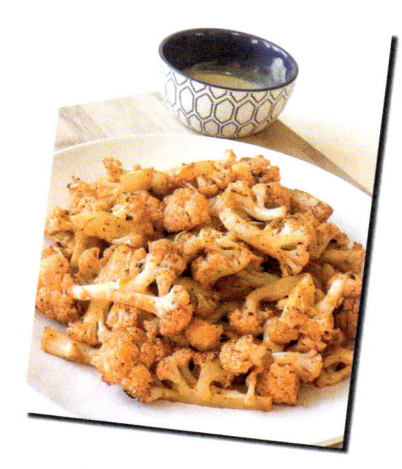

Nutritional Data (estimates) - per serving:
Calories: 189   Fat: 18 g   Total Carbs: 8 g   Fiber: 4 g   Sugar: 4 g   Net Carbs: 4 g   Protein: 3 g

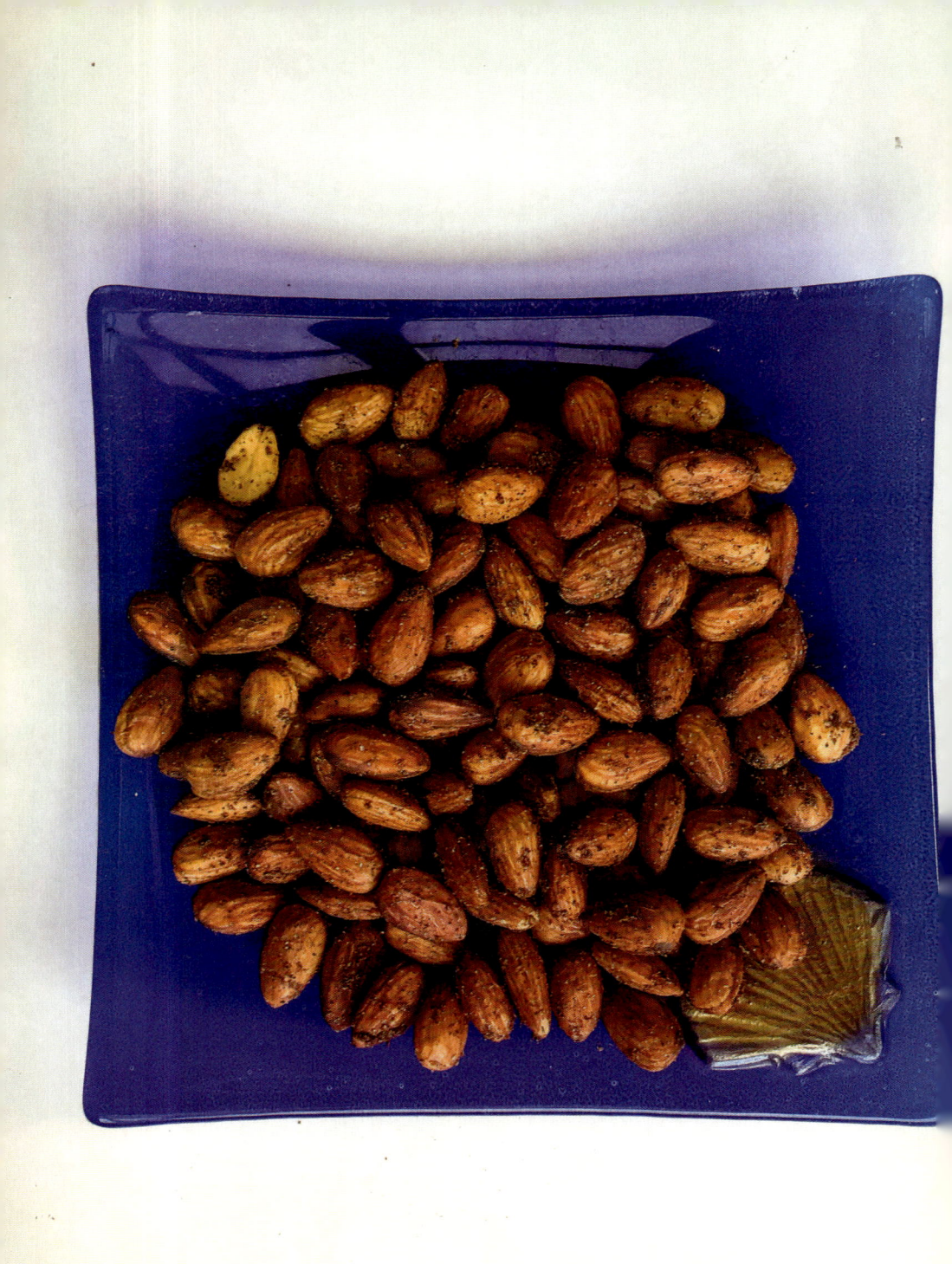

Cajun Roasted Almonds

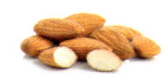

Prep Time: 5 minutes
Cook Time: 30 minutes
Yield: 4 servings

INGREDIENTS

- 2 cups (10 oz or 280 g) raw almonds (or other nuts of your choosing)
- 2 Tablespoons (30 ml) avocado oil
- 1 Tablespoon (6 g) paprika
- 2 teaspoons (7 g) garlic powder
- 1 teaspoon (3 g) onion powder
- 1 teaspoon (2 g) black pepper
- 1 teaspoon (2 g) cayenne pepper
- 2 teaspoons (10 g) salt

INSTRUCTIONS

1. Preheat oven to 300 F (150 C).

2. Toss the almonds with the avocado oil, spices, and salt in a small mixing bowl.

3. Place almonds on a parchment paper-lined baking tray and bake for 30 minutes until slightly browned.

4. Let cool and store in airtight container.

Nutritional Data (estimates) - per serving:
Calories: 175   Fat: 18 g   Total Carbs: 7 g   Fiber: 3 g   Sugar: 0 g   Net Carbs: 4 g   Protein: 5 g

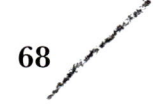

Bacon Stuffed Mushrooms

Prep Time: 10 minutes
Cook Time: 25 minutes
Yield: 4 servings

INGREDIENTS

- 20 medium white button mushrooms
- 4 slices of bacon, raw
- 1/4 onion
- 2 Tablespoons (30 ml) olive oil or avocado oil

INSTRUCTIONS

1. Preheat oven to 400 F (200 C).

2. Clean the mushrooms (remove the stems carefully with your hands – they should pop and then come out cleanly after you wriggle it a bit).

3. In the food processor, food process the bacon, onion, and mushroom stems to form a mince.

4. Heat up a frying pan, add in the oil and fry the mince until slightly browned.

5. Using your hands and a small spoon, stuff the bacon mixture into the mushrooms.

6. Place mushrooms onto a baking tray and bake for 15-20 minutes until slightly browned.

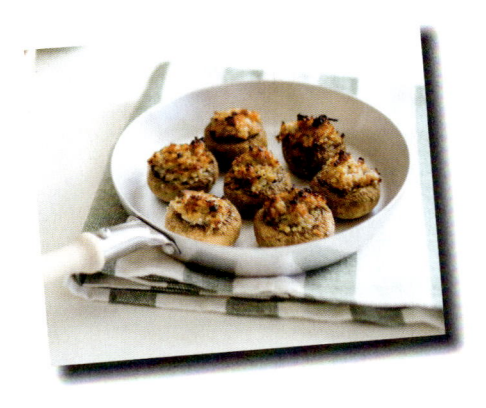

Nutritional Data (estimates) - per serving:
Calories: 200   Fat: 20 g   Total Carbs: 2 g   Fiber: 1 g   Sugar: 1 g   Net Carbs: 1 g   Protein: 5 g

Bacon & Chicken Omelet Bites

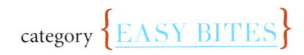

Prep Time: 15 minutes
Cook Time: 30 minutes
Yield: 12 servings

INGREDIENTS

- 1 chicken breast (1/2 lb or 225 g), diced
- 12 slices of bacon, cooked and broken into bits
- 8 eggs, whisked
- 1 medium bell pepper, diced
- 1/2 medium onion, diced

INSTRUCTIONS

1. Preheat oven to 350 F (175 C).

2. Line a muffin tray with liners or grease well or use a silicone muffin tray.

3. Cook the bacon and then cook the diced chicken breast in the leftover bacon fat. Let cool for a few minutes.

4. In a large bowl, combine the whisked eggs, bell pepper, onion, cooked chicken and bacon together.

5. Spoon the mixture into the muffin trays (makes 12 muffins) and bake for 30 minutes.

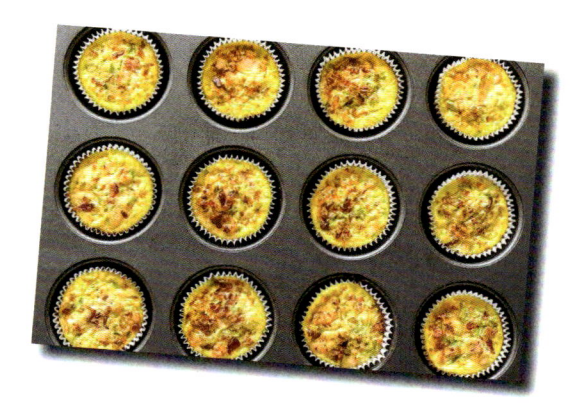

Nutritional Data (estimates) - per serving:
Calories: 206   Fat: 17 g   Total Carbs: 1 g   Fiber: 0 g   Sugar: 0 g   Net Carbs: 1 g   Protein: 11 g

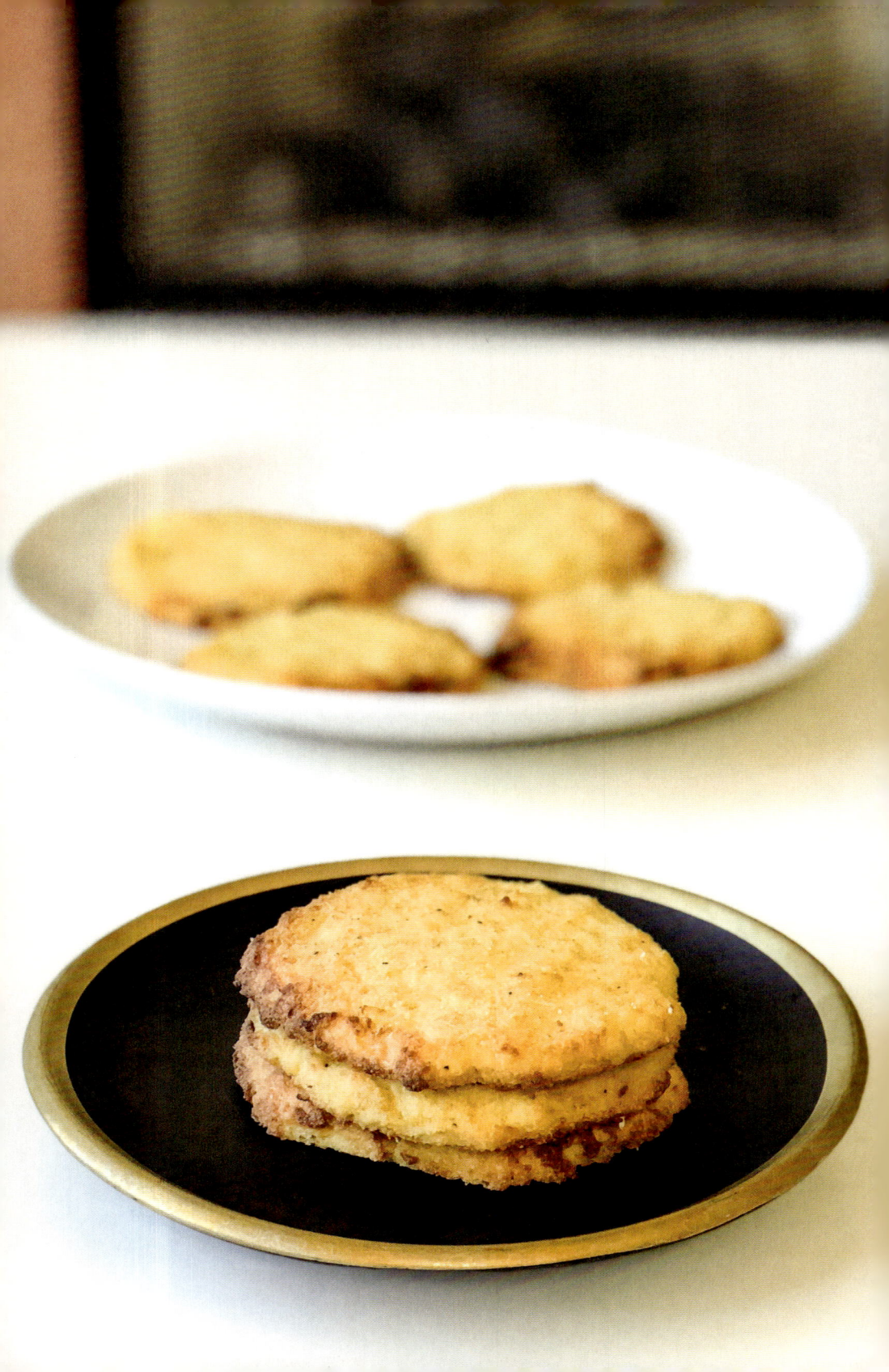

category { EASY BITES }

Cauliflower Patties

Prep Time: 10 minutes
Cook Time: 45 minutes
Yield: 4 servings

INGREDIENTS

- 1 head (approx. 1.5 lb or 600 g) cauliflower, broken into florets
- 2 eggs, whisked
- 1 cup (120 g) almond flour
- 1 Tablespoon (15 ml) coconut oil, for greasing baking tray
- Salt and pepper, to taste

INSTRUCTIONS

1. Preheat oven to 350 F (175 C).

2. Steam the cauliflower florets until softened.

3. Drain well and then food process or blend the cauliflower with the eggs and almond flour. Season with salt and pepper.

4. Form 8 patties. Place on a greased baking tray and bake for 30 minutes until slightly browned.

Nutritional Data (estimates) - per serving:
Calories: 234   Fat: 18 g   Total Carbs: 13 g   Fiber: 7 g   Sugar: 5 g   Net Carbs: 6 g   Protein: 11 g

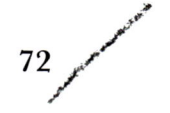

Mexican Lime and Chili Cucumbers

Prep Time: 2 minutes
Cook Time: 0 minutes
Yield: 4 servings

INGREDIENTS

- 2 large cucumbers, cut into large wedges (best chilled)
- 1/4 cup (56 g) cashews
- 3 Tablespoons (45 ml) olive oil
- Zest and juice of 1 lime
- 1 teaspoon (2 g) chili powder
- Salt and pepper, to taste

INSTRUCTIONS

1. Toss all the ingredients together.

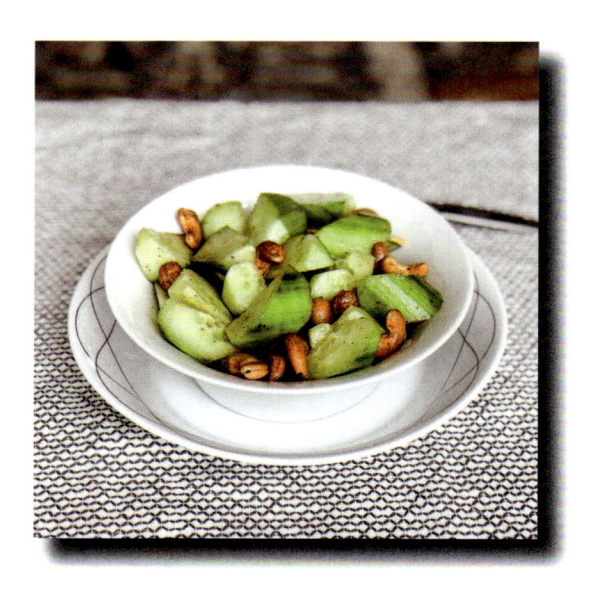

Nutritional Data (estimates) - per serving:
Calories: 151   Fat: 14 g   Total Carbs: 5 g   Fiber: 1 g   Sugar: 2 g   Net Carbs: 4 g   Protein: 3 g

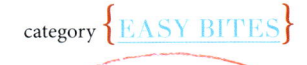
Fried "Spaghetti" Fritters

Prep Time: 15 minutes
Cook Time: 10 minutes
Yield: 8 servings

INGREDIENTS

- 1/2 large spaghetti squash (3 lb or 1.5 kg), seeds removed
- 2 eggs, whisked
- 3 Tablespoons (45 ml) olive oil
- 1 Tablespoon (3 g) Italian seasoning
- 1 Tablespoon (10 g) garlic powder
- 1 Tablespoon (7 g) onion powder
- Salt and black pepper, to taste

INSTRUCTIONS

1. Soften the spaghetti squash by placing it on a microwaveable plate (cover with a paper towel) and microwaving it for 8 minutes on high. When softened, you should be able to remove the strands easily with a fork. You can also bake the spaghetti squash, but it takes a lot longer to soften.

2. Remove the flesh and let cool for a few minutes before mixing with the eggs and all the seasoning.

3. Add the olive oil to a large frying pan over medium heat.

4. Using a large spoon, scoop squash mixture into the skillet and flatten slightly (makes approx. 8 fritters). Cook for 3 minutes then carefully turn and cook for another 2-3 minutes.

5. Remove from pan and drain on paper towels. Enjoy.

Nutritional Data (estimates) - per serving:
Calories: 82   Fat: 6 g   Total Carbs: 5 g   Fiber: 1 g   Sugar: 2 g   Net Carbs: 4 g   Protein: 2 g

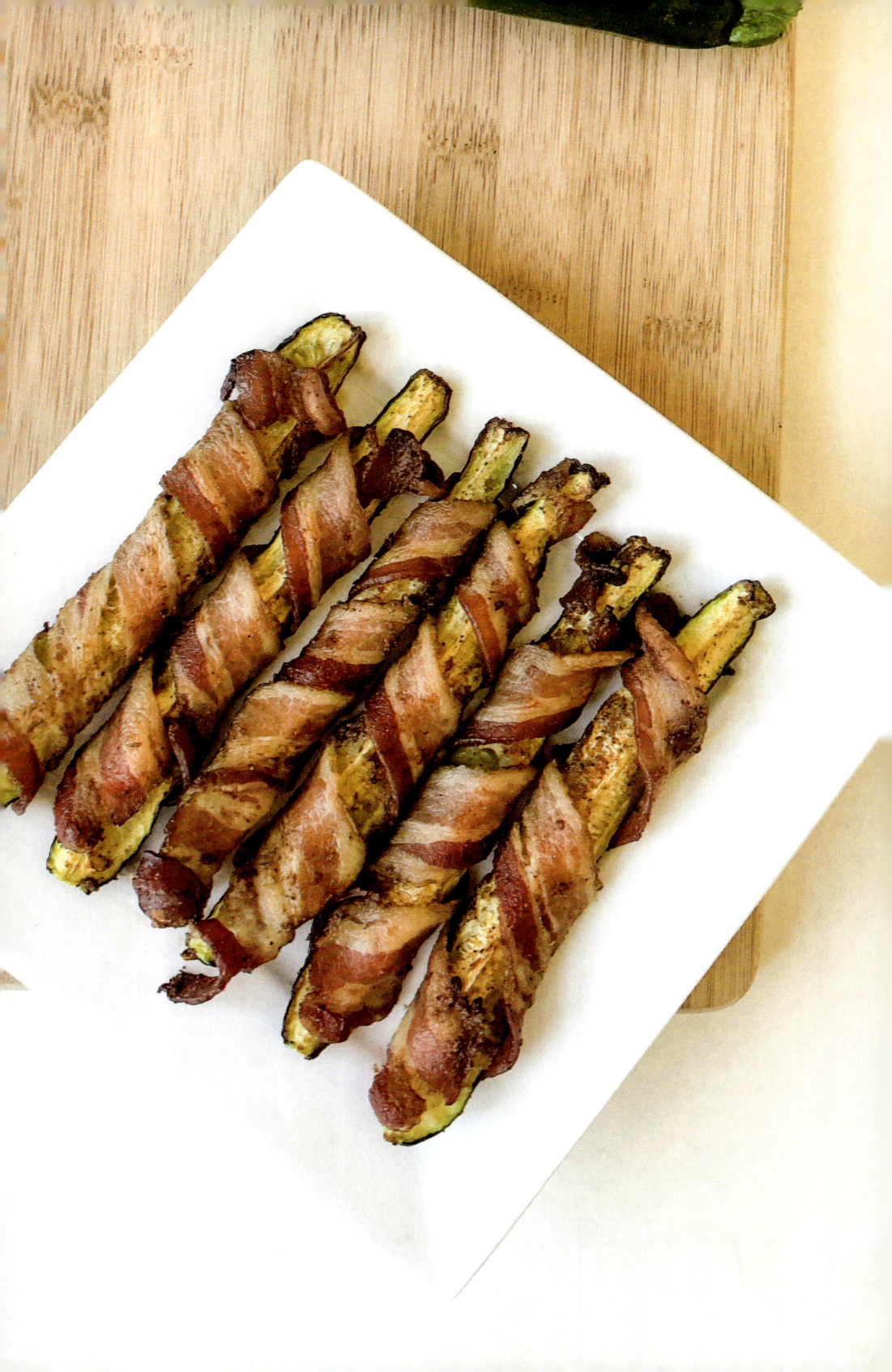

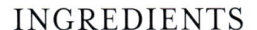
Zucchini Bacon Bites

Prep Time: 5 minutes
Cook Time: 35 minutes
Yield: 4 servings

INGREDIENTS
- 2 zucchinis, cut into 8 strips
- 8 thin slices of bacon, raw
- 2 Tablespoons (30 ml) olive oil
- 1 teaspoon (2 g) chili powder
- 1 teaspoon (3 g) garlic powder
- Salt and pepper, to taste

INSTRUCTIONS
1. Preheat oven to 350 F (175 C).
2. Place the zucchini strips into large mixing bowl and toss with olive oil, chili powder, garlic powder, salt and pepper.
3. Wrap a slice of bacon around each zucchini strip and place on a parchment paper-lined baking tray.
4. Bake for 35 minutes.
5. If you want the bacon crisper, place under the broiler for 3-5 minutes. Remove from oven and let cool slightly before serving.

Nutritional Data (estimates) - per serving:
Calories: 325   Fat: 33 g   Total Carbs: 2 g   Fiber: 1 g   Sugar: 1 g   Net Carbs: 1 g   Protein: 7 g

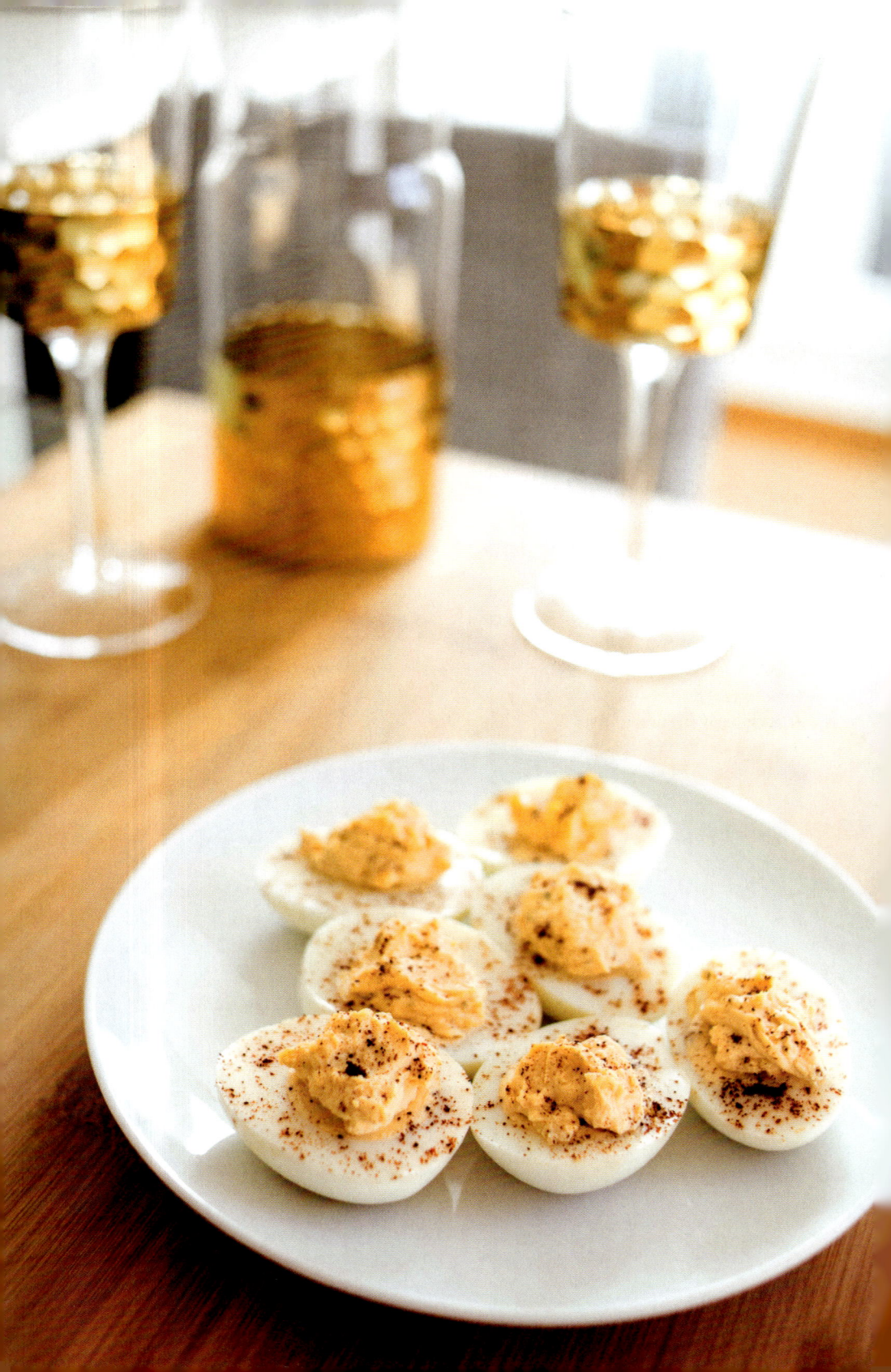

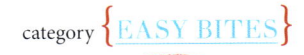

Paprika Deviled Eggs

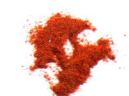

Prep Time: 5 minutes
Cook Time: 10 minutes
Yield: 4 servings

INGREDIENTS

- 8 eggs
- 1/4 cup (60 ml) mayo
- 2 teaspoons (10 ml) mustard
- 1 teaspoon (5 ml) lemon juice or white wine vinegar
- 1 teaspoon (2 g) smoked paprika, for sprinkling
- Salt and pepper, to taste

INSTRUCTIONS

1. Hard boil the eggs.

2. Slice in half lengthwise with a sharp knife.

3. Carefully remove the egg yolks and mash them with mayo, mustard, lemon juice or vinegar, salt, and pepper.

4. Spoon the mixture back into the egg whites.

5. Sprinkle with smoked paprika.

Nutritional Data (estimates) - per serving:
Calories: 226 Fat: 20 g Total Carbs: 0 g Fiber: 0 g Sugar: 0 g Net Carbs: 0 g Protein: 12 g

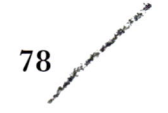

Smokey Bacon Meatballs

Prep Time: 15 minutes
Cook Time: 30 minutes
Yield: 8 servings

INGREDIENTS

- 2 chicken breasts or 1 lb (450 g) ground chicken
- 8 slices of bacon, cooked and crumbled
- 1 egg, whisked
- 2 cloves of garlic, peeled
- 1 Tablespoon (7 g) onion powder
- 2 drops of liquid smoke
- 4 Tablespoons (60 ml) avocado or olive oil, to cook with

INSTRUCTIONS

1. Place everything (except the oil) into a food processor and mix well.

2. From the mixture, form 20-24 small meatballs.

3. Place the oil into a large frying pan, and fry the meatballs until the meat is cooked (cook one side for 5 minutes until browned, then flip and cook the other side for 5-10 minutes until done). You will probably need to cook them in a few batches.

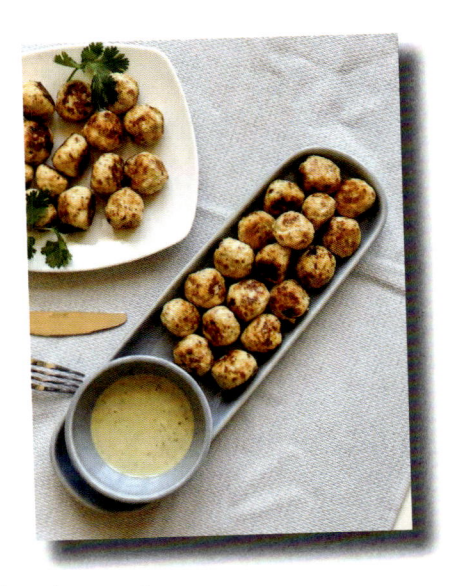

Nutritional Data (estimates) - per serving:
Calories: 279   Fat: 25 g   Total Carbs: 1 g   Fiber: 0 g   Sugar: 0 g   Net Carbs: 1 g   Protein: 13 g

Chapter 6:
Delicacies

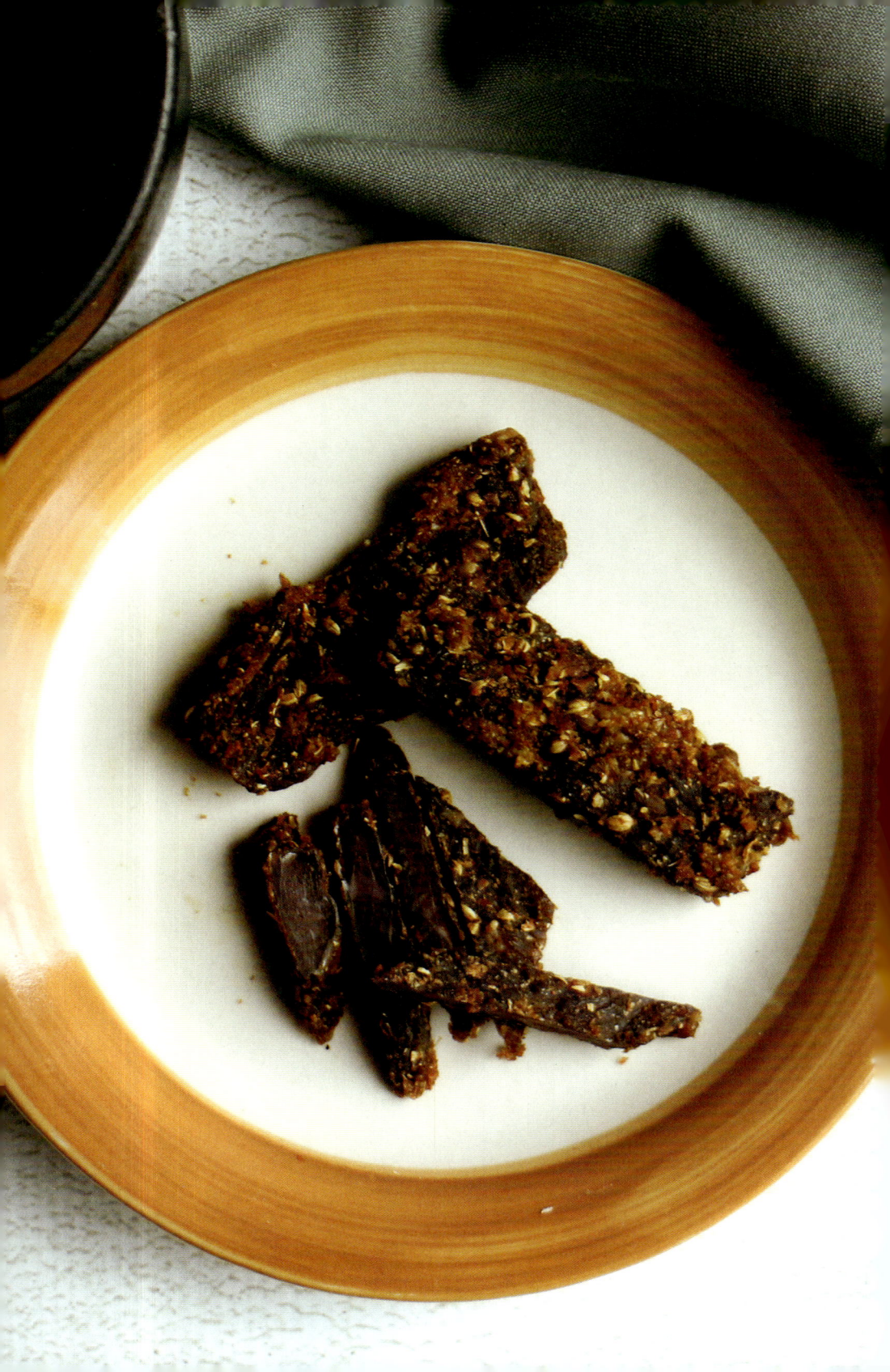

Beef Jerky

Prep Time: 10 minutes + overnight
Cook Time: 8-10 hours
Yield: approx. 35 servings

INGREDIENTS

- 2.2 lbs (1 kg) of beef roast, fat trimmed
- 1/4 cup (60 ml) vinegar of your choice
- 2 Tablespoons (14 g) onion powder
- 2 Tablespoons (20 g) garlic powder
- 1 teaspoon (1 g) ground coriander
- 2 Tablespoons (30 g) salt
- 1 Tablespoon (1 g) coriander seeds, crushed
- 3 Tablespoons (45 ml) gluten-free tamari sauce or coconut aminos
- Black pepper, to taste

INSTRUCTIONS

1. Cut beef into 1-inch thick pieces along the grain. Pour vinegar into a bowl then dip each piece of raw meat in it. Allow the excess vinegar to stop dripping, then place the piece on a cooling rack set over a tray. Place the uncovered tray in the fridge overnight.

2. In a bowl, combine the onion powder, garlic powder, ground coriander, and salt, plus a generous sprinkle of black pepper. Partially crush the coriander seeds using a pestle and mortar and add to the mixture. Add the tamari sauce to form a paste.

3. Pat dry the meat then add to the bowl of paste. Massage the paste into each piece of meat.

4. Lay the pieces on a dehydrator set at 140 F (60 C) for 8-10 hours, depending on how moist you like the jerky. Turn them over occasionally.

5. Store in a sealed container.

Nutritional Data (estimates) - per serving:
Calories: 79   Fat: 6 g   Total Carbs: 1 g   Fiber: 0 g   Sugar: 0 g   Net Carbs: 1 g   Protein: 5 g

Baked Scotch Eggs

Prep Time: 15 minutes
Cooking Time: 30 minutes
Yield: 6 servings

INGREDIENTS

- 6 hard-boiled eggs, peeled
- 1 lb (450 g) ground pork sausage with casings removed (or use ground pork with 1 Tablespoon (3 g) Italian seasoning)
- 1/4 cup (30 g) almond flour
- 2 Tablespoons (14 g) flax or chia seeds, ground into a meal (use a food processor, blender, or coffee grinder)
- 2 Tablespoons (30 ml) olive or avocado oil
- Salt and black pepper, to taste

INSTRUCTIONS

1. Preheat oven to 350 F (175 C).

2. In a small bowl, stir together the pork, almond flour, flax/chia meal, olive oil, salt and pepper.

3. Divide the meat mixture into 6 portions and flatten into patties and wrap around the boiled eggs, covering each egg completely. (Add additional olive oil or a bit of water to help the mixture stick together if needed.) Use some plastic wrap to help you get the mixture tightly around the boiled eggs.

4. Place on parchment paper-lined baking trays and bake for 15 minutes. Then turn the eggs over carefully and bake for another 15 minutes, or until sausage is cooked through. Remove from oven and let cool.

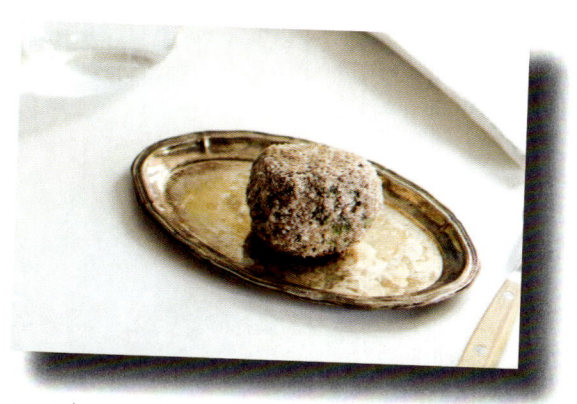

Nutritional Data (estimates) - per serving:
Calories: 198   Fat: 11 g   Total Carbs: 2 g   Fiber: 1 g   Sugar: 0 g   Net Carbs: 1 g   Protein: 24 g

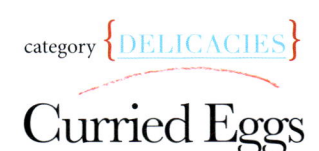

Curried Eggs

Prep Time: 15 minutes
Cook Time: 5 minutes
Yield: 3 servings

INGREDIENTS

- 6 eggs
- 2 Tablespoons (30 ml) coconut oil, to cook with
- 2 cloves of garlic, peeled and minced
- 1 Tablespoon (7 g) curry powder
- 1 teaspoon (5 g) salt or to taste

INSTRUCTIONS

1. Hard boil the eggs.
2. Make a few slits in the eggs.
3. Place the coconut oil into a frying pan on medium heat.
4. Add in the garlic, curry powder, salt, and the eggs.
5. Fry for 2-3 minutes until the eggs are coated in the curry mixture.

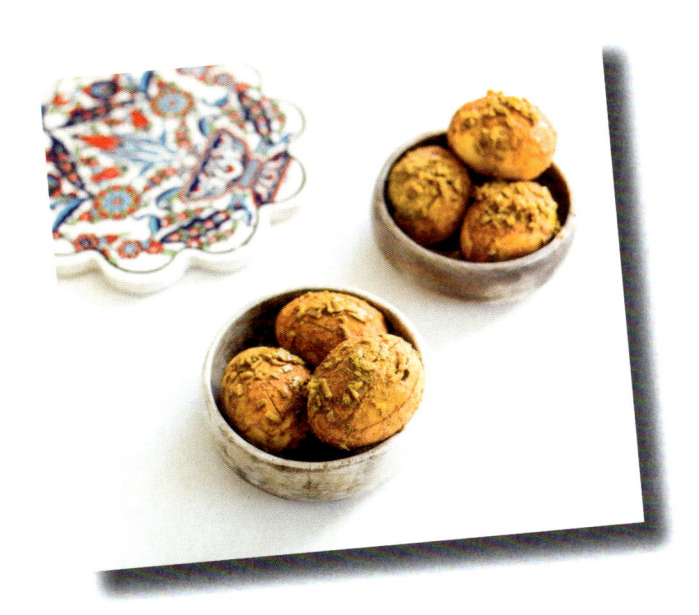

Nutritional Data (estimates) - per serving:
Calories: 215   Fat: 17 g   Total Carbs: 2 g   Fiber: 1 g   Sugar: 0 g   Net Carbs: 1 g   Protein: 12 g

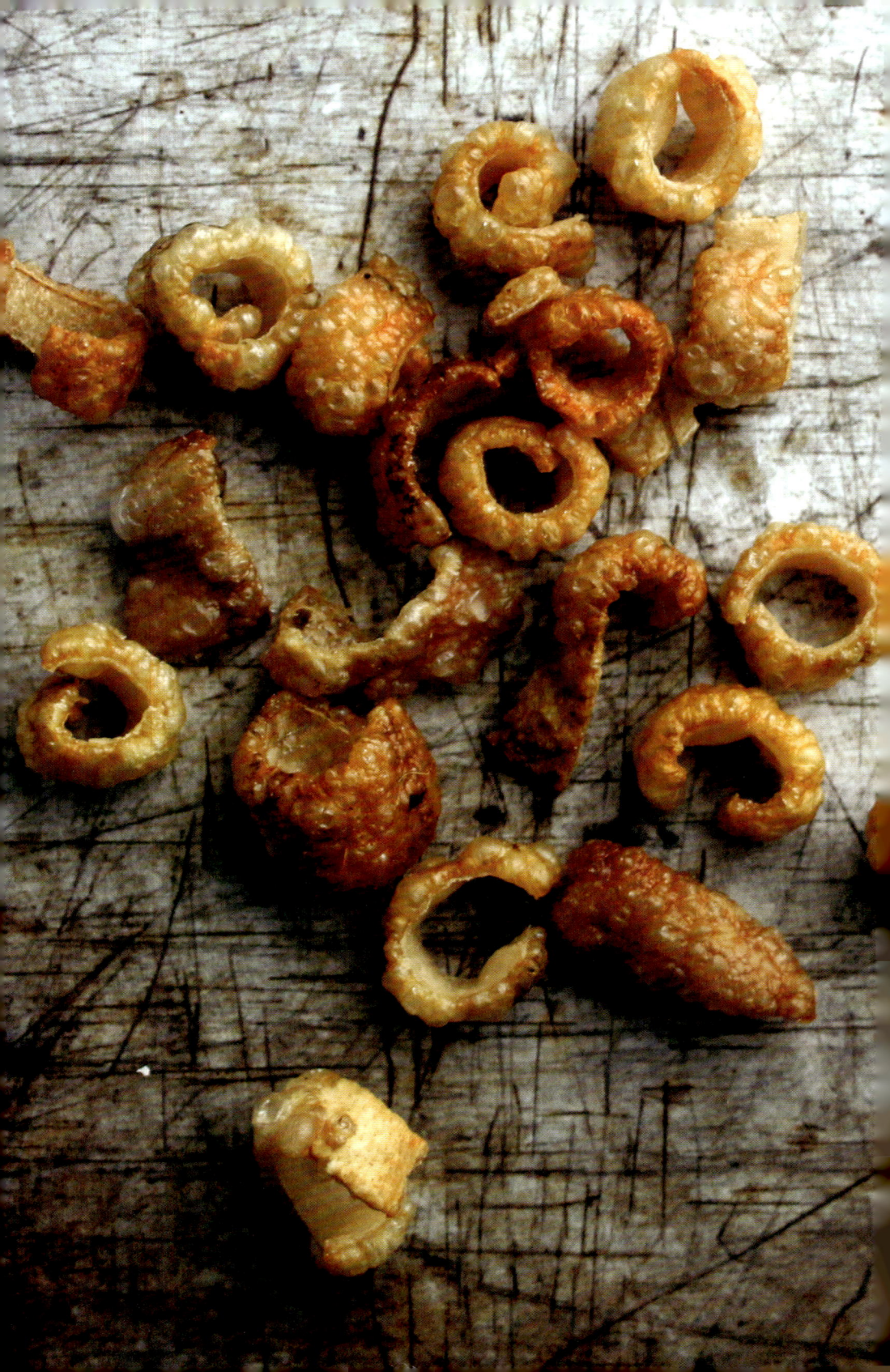

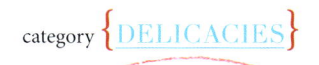

Basic Pork Rind

Prep Time: 20 minutes
Cook Time: 2 hours 10 minutes
Yield: 4 servings

INGREDIENTS

- 1 large piece of pork skin (approx. 2.2 lbs or 1 kg)
- Salt and spices of choice (suggestion – Chinese five spices)

INSTRUCTIONS

1. Preheat the oven to 250 F (120 C). If your oven doesn't go down to this low of a temperature, set it to its lowest temperature and then open the oven door a crack.
2. Use a very sharp knife to remove all the fat from the skin.
3. You should be left with only the transparent skin.
4. Pat both sides dry and trim into smaller pieces (approx. 1-inch by 1-inch).
5. Salt the pieces well and place on a wire rack placed over a tray. Place in the oven for 2 hours to dry out.
6. Remove the tray from the oven and transfer the pieces onto a clean tray.
7. Increase the temperature of the oven to max 440 F (230 C).
8. Once at temperature, place the tray into the oven and cook for 5-10 minutes allowing them to pop. (Alternatively, you can pop the pork rinds by shallow frying them for 3-5 minutes in olive oil, lard, coconut oil, avocado oil.)
9. Season with salt and spices of your choosing.
10. Allow to cool completely before storing in a sealed container. Makes approx. 30-50 pieces.

Nutritional Data (estimates) - per serving:
Calories: 152   Fat: 9 g   Total Carbs: 0 g   Fiber: 0 g   Sugar: 0 g   Net Carbs: 0 g Protein: 17 g

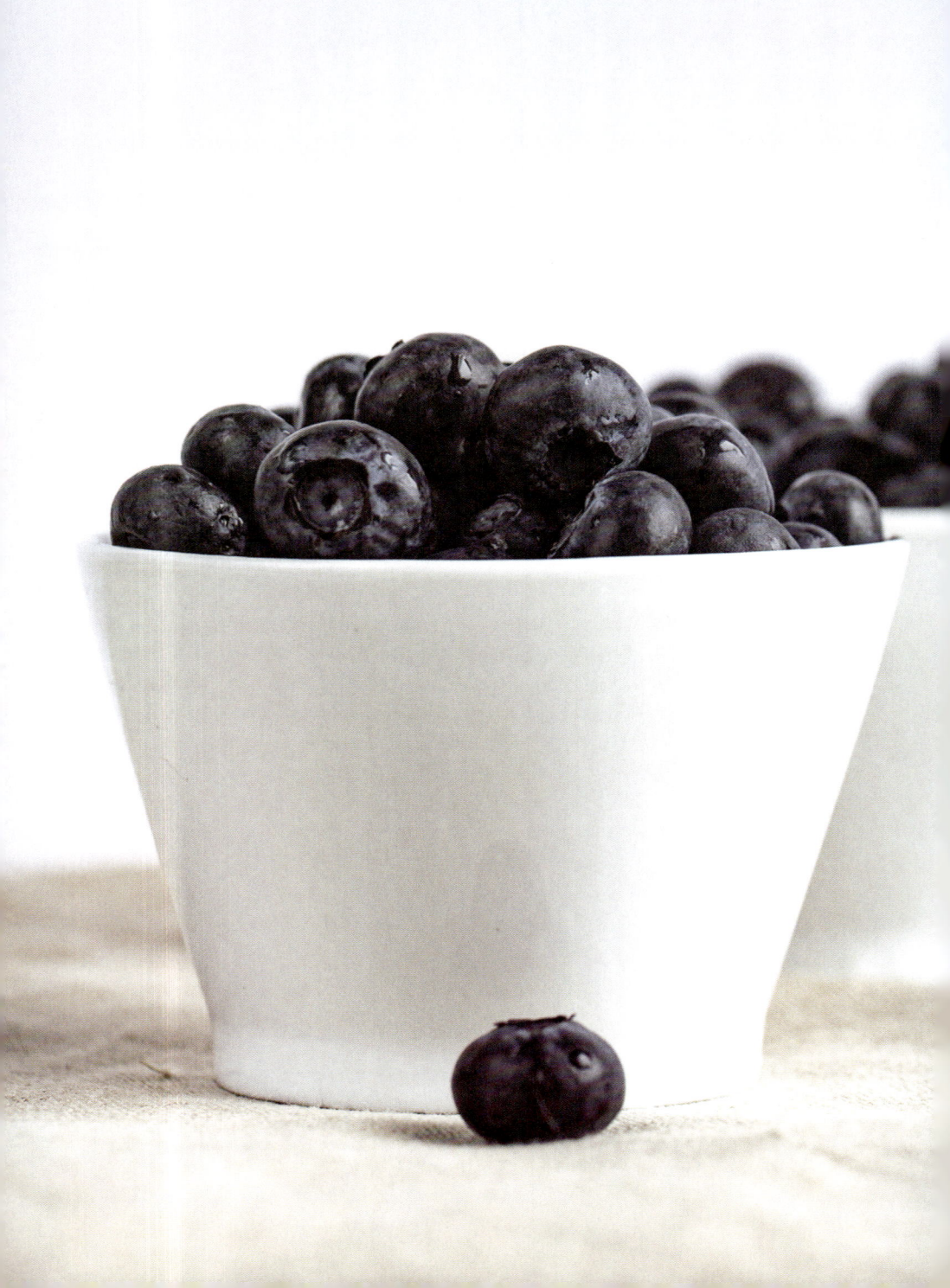

Chapter 7:
Frozen Delights

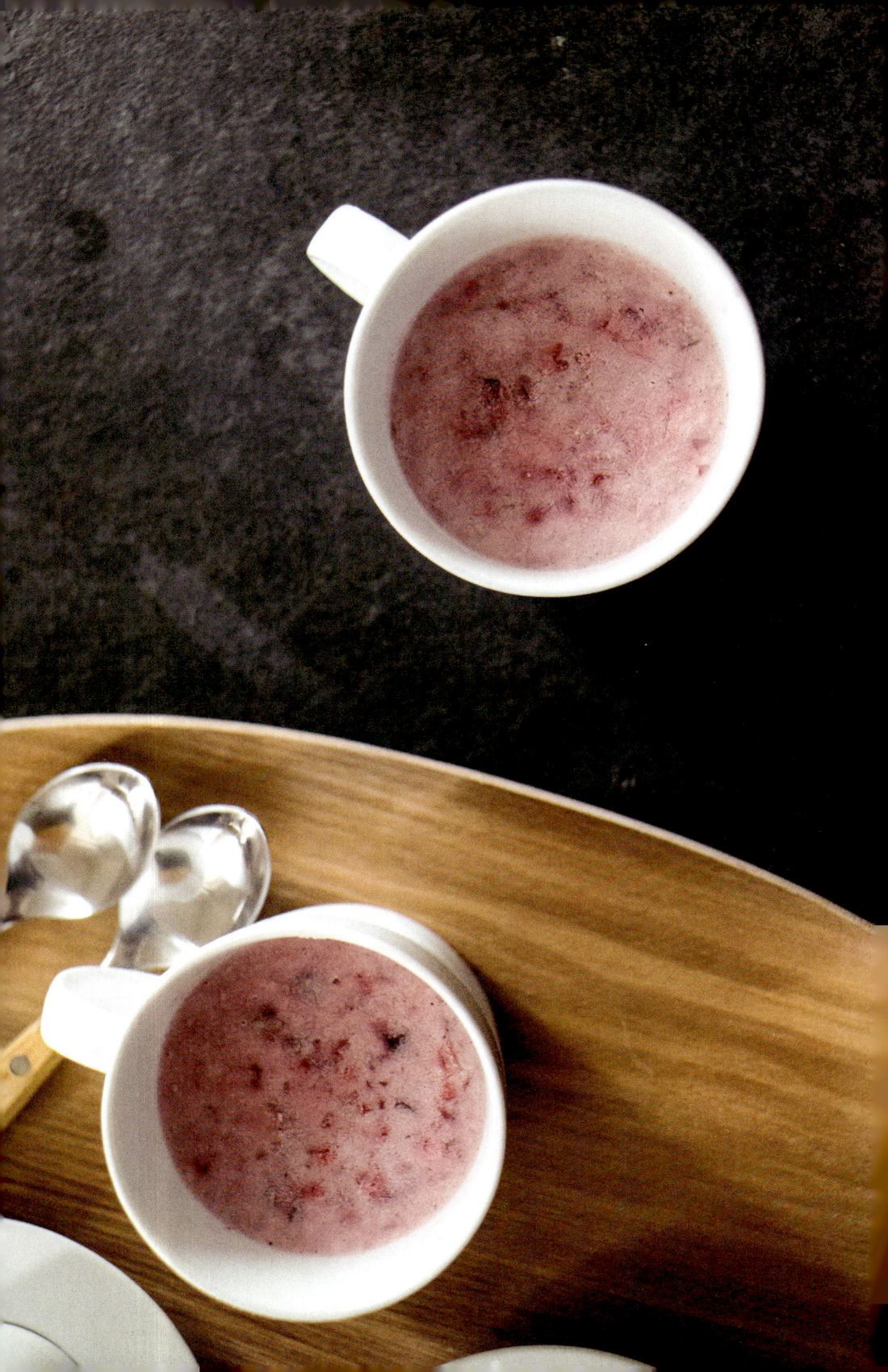

Berry Frozen "Yogurt"

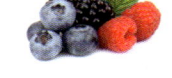

Prep Time: 5 minutes
Freezing Time: 30 minutes + 2 hours
Yield: 6 servings

INGREDIENTS

- 1 cup (70 g) mixed berries
- 1 cup (240 ml) coconut cream (from the top of refrigerated cans of coconut milk)
- 1 teaspoon (5 ml) vanilla extract
- Zest and juice of 1/2 lemon
- 2 Tablespoons (24 g) erythritol or stevia, to taste

INSTRUCTIONS

1. Mix together the vanilla, coconut cream, lemon, erythritol or stevia and freeze for 30 minutes.

2. Food process or blend the frozen coconut cream mixture and berries (for a few pulses).

3. Divide between 6 small containers/glasses.

4. Place back into the freezer and freeze for 2+ hours. You may need to thaw it a bit before serving.

Nutritional Data (estimates) - per serving:
Calories: 117 Fat: 8 g Total Carbs: 10 g Fiber: 5 g Sugar: 4 g Net Carbs: 5 g Protein: 0 g

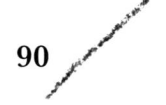

Blueberry Popsicles

Prep Time: 10 minutes
Freezing Time: 4+ hours
Yield: 2 servings

INGREDIENTS

- 1/4 cup blueberries
- 1/2 cup (120 ml) coconut milk
- Stevia or erythritol, to taste
- 1 Tablespoon (15 ml) lemon juice
- 1 teaspoon (5 ml) vanilla extract

INSTRUCTIONS

1. Blend all the ingredients together well.

2. Taste the mixture and add more of any ingredient you want.

3. Pour into ice pop molds (this recipe makes approx. two 2.5 oz bars). Make sure there's a bit of space left over as the mixture will expand when it freezes.

4. Freeze for 4+ hours. When ready to eat, run the ice pop mold for a few minutes under hot water to make it easier to pull the ice pops out.

Nutritional Data (estimates) - per serving:
Calories: 112   Fat: 11 g   Total Carbs: 4 g   Fiber: 1 g   Sugar: 2 g   Net Carbs: 3 g   Protein: 1 g

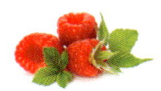

Frozen Chocolate Berries

Prep Time: 5 minutes
Freezing Time: 2+ hours
Yield: 2 servings

INGREDIENTS
- 1 oz (30 g) 100% chocolate
- 5 raspberries
- 10 blueberries
- 1 teaspoon (5 ml) of almond butter (optional)

INSTRUCTIONS
1. Melt the dark chocolate in the microwave. This usually takes around 1 1/2 to 2 minutes.

2. Pour the chocolate into 2 muffin liners in a muffin tin.

3. Place the berries into the melted chocolate.

4. Finish by drizzling the almond butter over the top of the berries and chocolate. (Makes 2 cups)

5. Freeze for 2+ hours.

Nutritional Data (estimates) - per serving:
Calories: 96   Fat: 4 g   Total Carbs: 5 g   Fiber: 2 g   Sugar: 2 g   Net Carbs: 3 g   Protein: 2 g

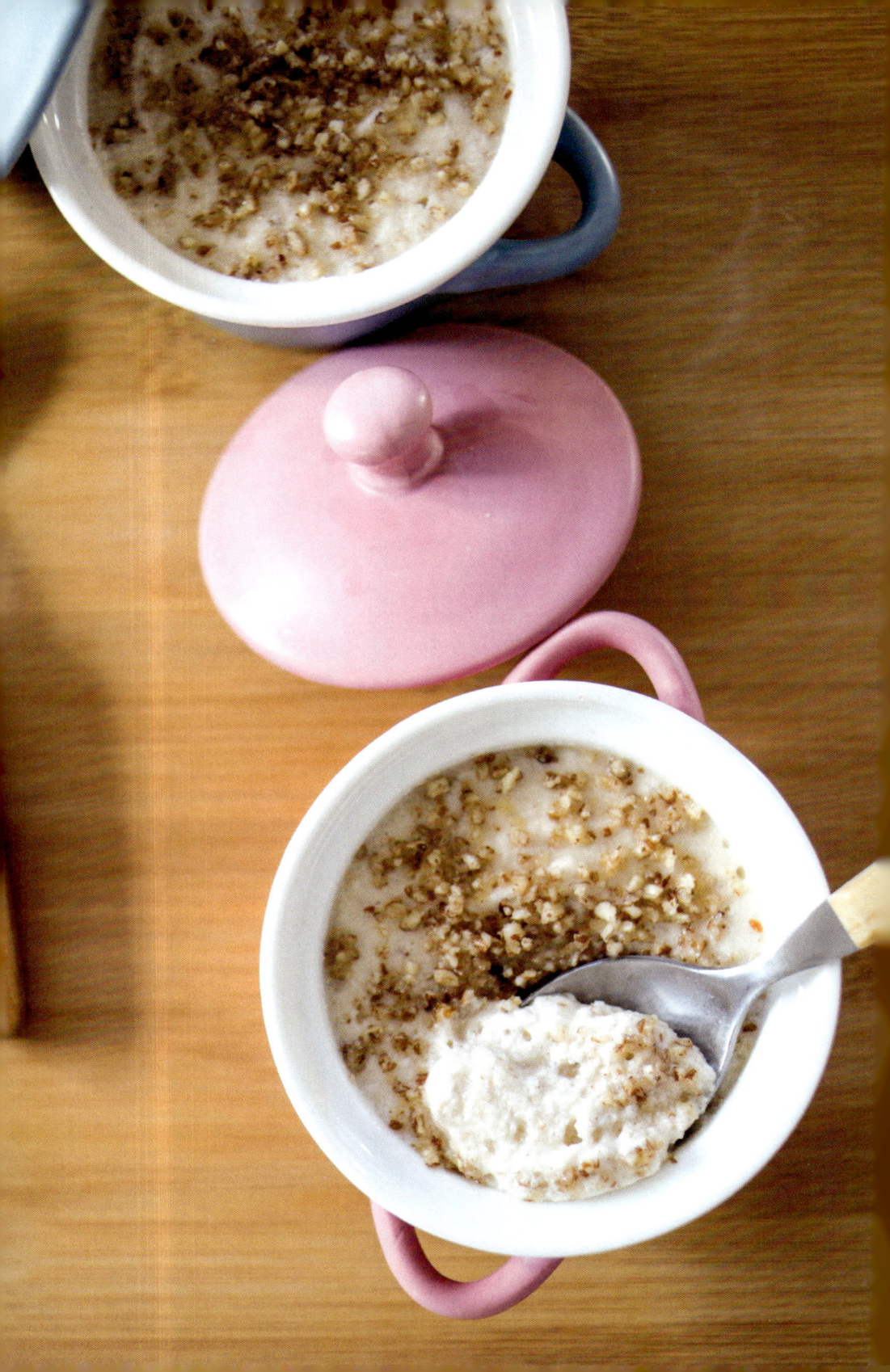

Vanilla Pecan Ice Cream

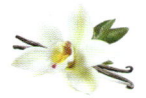

Prep Time: 15 minutes
Freezing Time: 2+ hours
Yield: 2 servings

INGREDIENTS

- 2 eggs
- 3 Tablespoons (36 g) erythritol (or to taste)
- 1/2 cup (120 ml) coconut cream (from the top of refrigerated cans of coconut milk)
- 2 Tablespoons (15 g) pecan pieces
- 2 teaspoons (10 ml) vanilla extract

INSTRUCTIONS

1. Separate the egg yolks from the whites.

2. Whisk the egg whites until they form stiff peaks. Whisk in the erythritol and coconut cream.

3. Then fold in the egg yolks, pecan pieces, and vanilla extract.

4. Pour into 2 small containers and freezer for 2+ hours.

Nutritional Data (estimates) - per serving:
Calories: 243   Fat: 22 g   Total Carbs: 3 g   Fiber: 2 g   Sugar: 1 g   Net Carbs: 1 g   Protein: 7 g

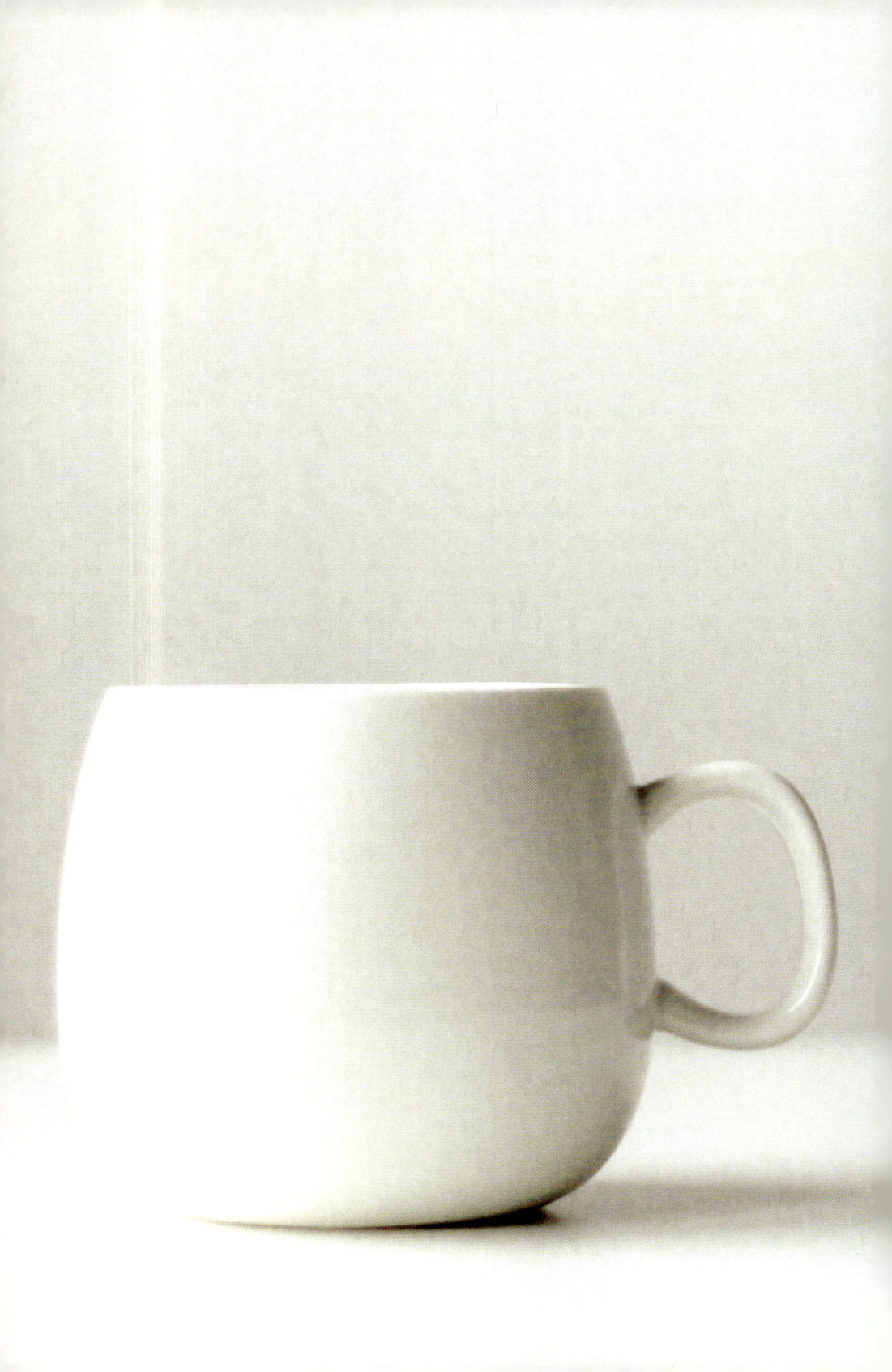

Chapter 8:
Other Desserts

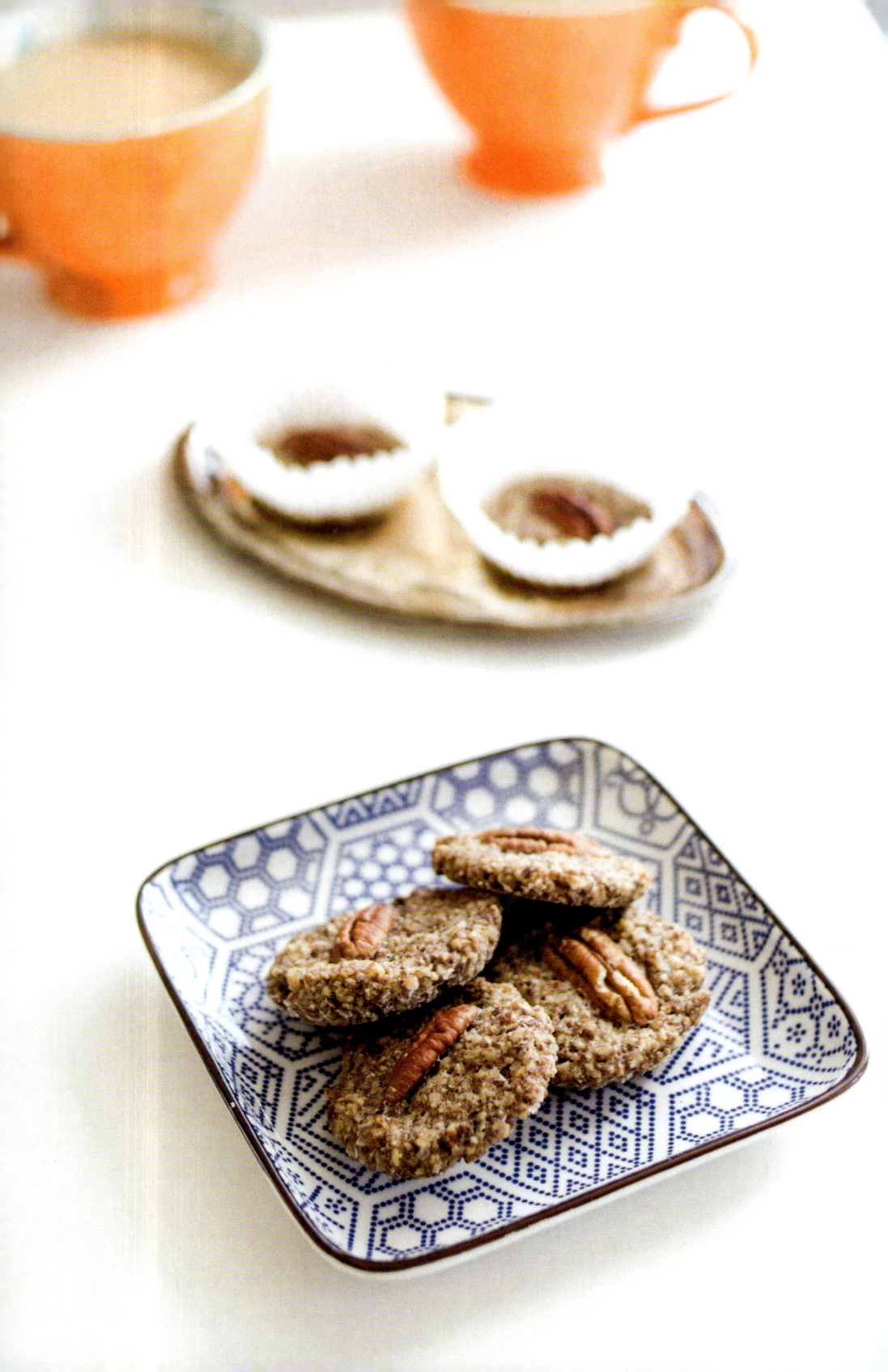

Pecan Crisps

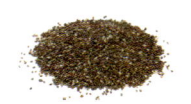

Prep Time: 10 minutes
Cook Time: 10 minutes
Yield: 6 servings

INGREDIENTS

- 1.5 cups (150 g) pecans, chopped
- 12 pecan halves (24 g), for topping
- 1/4 cup (48 g) erythritol or stevia, to taste
- 1 egg, whisked
- 1/4 cup (30 g) flax or chia seed, ground into a meal in a blender or food processor or coffee grinder

INSTRUCTIONS

1. Preheat oven to 350 F (175 C).

2. Food process the 1.5 cups of pecans, erythritol, egg, and flax/chia meal together.

3. Place 12 muffin liners into a muffin pan.

4. Divide the mixture between the 12 muffin liners.

5. Bake for 8-10 minutes. Press a pecan half on top of each pecan crisp.

6. Remove from oven and let cool slightly before storing in an airtight container.

Nutritional Data (estimates) - per serving:
Calories: 170   Fat: 14 g   Total Carbs: 7 g   Fiber: 4 g   Sugar: 1 g   Net Carbs: 3 g   Protein: 7 g

Chocolate Fudge

Prep Time: 10 minutes
Freezer Time: 1 hour
Yield: 12 servings

INGREDIENTS

- 4 oz (112 g) 100% dark chocolate
- 3/4 cup (175 ml) coconut butter
- 1 teaspoon (5 ml) vanilla extract
- Stevia or erythritol, to taste

INSTRUCTIONS

1. Melt the chocolate.

2. Melt the coconut butter.

3. Combine all the ingredients together in a bowl with a fork.

4. Pour into a silicone loaf pan or a parchment paper-lined pan.

5. Place into the fridge for 2+ hours or freezer for 1 hour until it's solidified.

6. Remove from the pan and cut into 12 pieces.

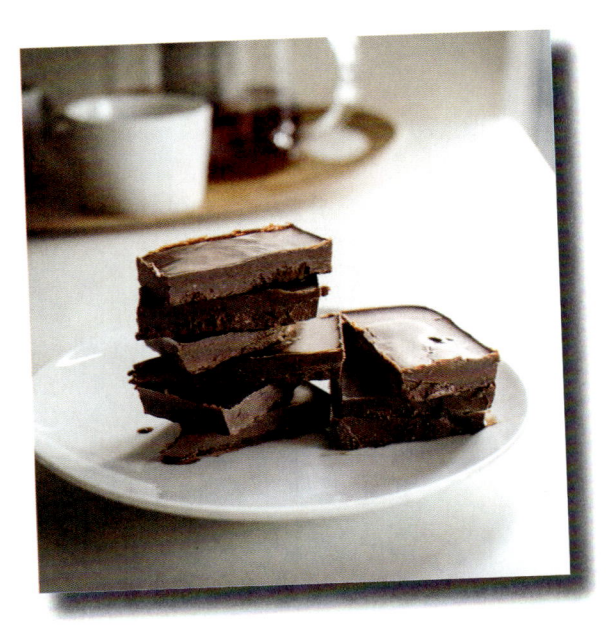

Nutritional Data (estimates) - per serving:
Calories: 158   Fat: 13 g   Total Carbs: 4 g   Fiber: 2 g   Sugar: 1 g   Net Carbs: 2 g   Protein: 2 g

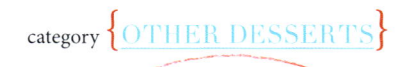

Coconut Butter Pecan Fat Bomb Bites

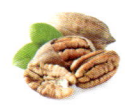

Prep Time: 10 minutes
Fridge Time: 20 minutes
Yield: 4 servings

INGREDIENTS

- 2 Tablespoons (30 g) coconut butter
- Dash of cinnamon powder
- Dash of ginger powder
- Dash of nutmeg powder
- Dash of cloves powder
- Stevia or erythritol, to taste
- 20 pecan halves (40 g)

INSTRUCTIONS

1. Warm the coconut butter so that it's softened.

2. Mix the coconut butter, cinnamon, ginger, nutmeg, cloves, and stevia together.

3. Using a teaspoon, place small scoops of the coconut butter mixture on top of each pecan half.

4. Place into the fridge to set for 20 minutes.

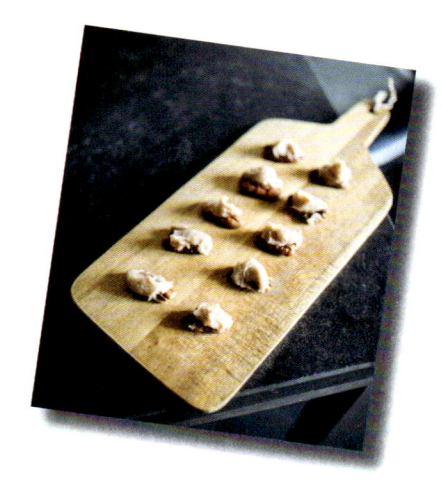

Nutritional Data (estimates) - per serving:
Calories: 160   Fat: 15 g   Total Carbs: 5 g   Fiber: 3 g   Sugar: 1 g   Net Carbs: 2 g   Protein: 2 g

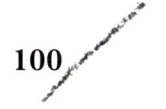

Mini Pecan Pies

Prep Time: 15 minutes
Cook Time: 15 minutes
Yield: 6 servings

INGREDIENTS

For the crust:

- 1/2 cup (60 g) almond flour
- 1 egg, whisked
- 2 Tablespoons (14 g) flax meal
- 2 Tablespoons (30 ml) ghee, melted but not too hot

For the filling:

- 1/2 cup (60 g) pecans, roughly chopped
- 1/4 cup (60 ml) ghee, melted but not too hot
- 1 egg, whisked
- 1/4 cup (48 g) granulated erythritol (or stevia)
- 1 teaspoon (5 ml) vanilla extract

INSTRUCTIONS

1. Preheat oven to 350 F (175 C).

2. Make the crust by mixing all the crust ingredients together. Press the dough into 6 mini muffin cups to form the crust.

3. Make the filling by mixing together all the filling ingredients in a bowl.

4. Pour into the 6 crusts.

5. Bake for 15 minutes until the pie crust is slightly golden.

6. Let cool then enjoy.

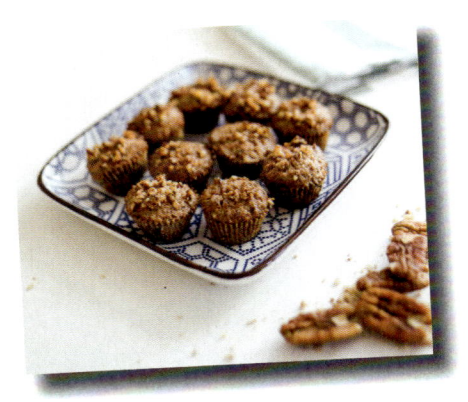

Nutritional Data (estimates) - per serving:
Calories: 243   Fat: 24 g   Total Carbs: 4 g   Fiber: 3 g   Sugar: 1 g   Net Carbs: 1 g   Protein: 6 g

Peppermint Patties

Prep Time: 15 minutes
Freezer Time: 3 hours
Yield: 12 servings

INGREDIENTS

To make the peppermint filling:

- 1/2 cup (120 ml) coconut butter
- 1 Tablespoon (15 ml) coconut oil, melted
- 1 teaspoon (5 ml) peppermint extract
- 1/4 cup (48 g) eryrithol or stevia, to taste

To make the chocolate layer:

- 2 Tablespoons (60 ml) coconut oil, melted
- 4 oz (112 g) 100% dark chocolate

INSTRUCTIONS

1. In a bowl mix together all the peppermint filling ingredients.

2. Pour a small amount of the peppermint mixture into mini cupcake or muffin trays (silicone ones work best for this) to form a 1/3-inch (0.8 cm) thick layer. Freeze for 1 hour until solid.

3. Melt the dark chocolate and coconut oil together and combine. Make sure it's not too hot but still liquid.

4. Remove the solid peppermint fillings from the cups.

5. Pour a small amount of the chocolate mixture into each cup so that it covers the base, place the peppermint filling back into the cup and then cover with a bit more chocolate so that it's completely covered. Repeat for all the patties (makes approx. 12 patties).

6. Freeze for 2+ hours until solid. Thaw for 10 minutes before enjoying.

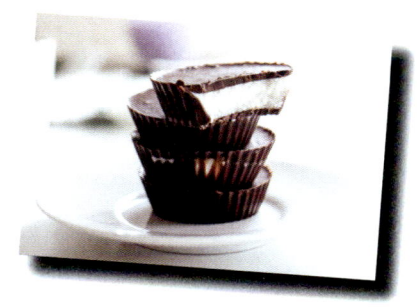

Nutritional Data (estimates) - per serving:
Calories: 153   Fat: 13 g   Total Carbs: 3 g   Fiber: 2 g   Sugar: 1 g   Net Carbs: 1 g   Protein: 2 g

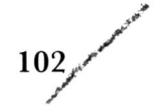

Lemon Drop Gummies

Prep Time: 15 minutes
Cook Time: 15 minutes
Yield: 4 servings

INGREDIENTS

- 1/4 cup (60 ml) fresh lemon juice
- 2 Tablespoons (12 g) gelatin powder
- 2 Tablespoons (24 g) erythritol or stevia, to taste

INSTRUCTIONS

1. In a small saucepan, heat up the lemon juice and slowly stir in the gelatin powder and erythritol so that it all dissolves.
2. Pour into silicone molds (or ice-cube trays).
3. Freeze or refrigerate for 2+ hours.

Nutritional Data (estimates) - per serving:
Calories: 15   Fat: 0 g   Total Carbs: 1 g   Fiber: 0 g   Sugar: 1 g   Net Carbs: 1 g   Protein: 3 g

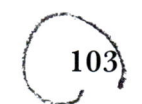

Jaffa Dark Chocolate Mousse

Prep Time: 10 minutes
Cook Time: 0 minutes
Yield: 6 servings

INGREDIENTS

- 2 ripe avocados (approx. 1 lb or 450 g), de-stoned and scoop out the flesh
- 3 Tablespoons (18 g) 100% cacao powder
- Zest of 1 navel orange
- Erythritol or stevia, to taste

INSTRUCTIONS

1. Blend everything together well. Taste the mousse and add more sweetener if needed.

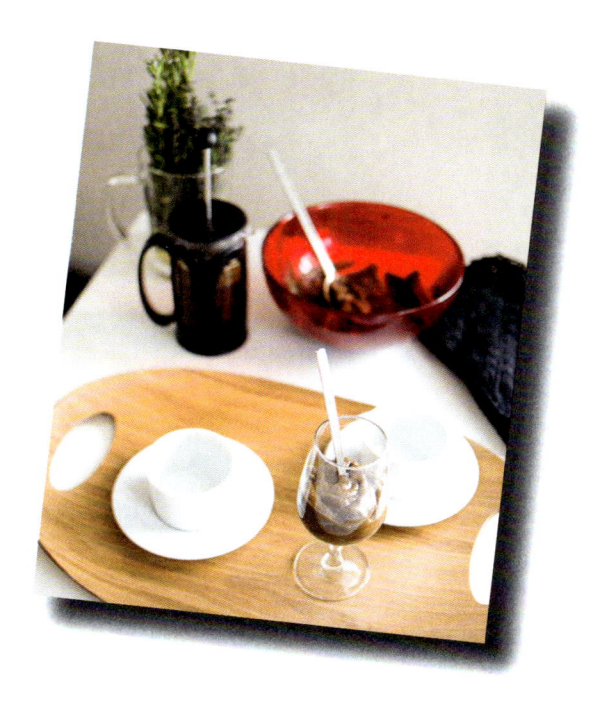

Nutritional Data (estimates) - per serving:
Calories: 119   Fat: 10 g   Total Carbs: 7 g   Fiber: 5 g   Sugar: 0 g   Net Carbs: 2 g   Protein: 2 g